Surgery
on the Move

Authors: Jenna Morgan, Harriet Walker
and Andrew Viggars
Editorial Advisors: Lynda Wyld, Jeff Garner,
Derek J. Rosario, Ahmed Nassef
and Anil Hormis
Series Editors: Rory Mackinnon, Sally Keat,
Thomas Locke and Andrew Walker

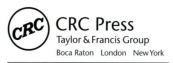

CRC Press
Taylor & Francis Group
Boca Raton London New York

CRC Press is an imprint of the
Taylor & Francis Group, an **informa** business

Cover images © Sebastian Kaulitzki—Fotolia & © franckreporter/istockphoto.com (smartphone)

First published in 2013 by
CRC Press
Taylor & Francis Group
6000 Broken Sound Parkway NW, Suite 300
Boca Raton, FL 33487-2742

© 2014 Morgan, Walker and Viggars
CRC Press is an imprint of Taylor & Francis Group, an Informa business
No claim to original U.S. Government works
Printed and bound in India by Replika Press Pvt. Ltd.
Version Date: 20120813
International Standard Book Number: 978-1-444-17601-8
1 2 3 4 5 6 7 8 9 10

**Visit the Taylor & Francis Web site at
http://www.taylorandfrancis.com
and the CRC Press Web site at
http://www.crcpress.com**

Contents

Preface

Have you ever found surgery bland or overwhelmingly complicated? Do you often forget the basics and then struggle with the core texts? Are you simply short of time and have exams looming? If so, then this short revision guide will help you. Written by students for students, this book presents information in a wide range of forms including flow charts, colourful diagrams, and summary tables. No matter what your learning style, this book is as appealing as it is easy to read. Its innovative style will help you learn and understand, and possibly even enjoy it, whilst also helping to bridge the gap to the recommended core texts.

Authors:

Jenna Morgan MBChB MRCSEd PGDipMedEd – ST3 in General Surgery, Yorkshire and Humber Deanery, Yorkshire, UK

Harriet Walker MBChB BMedSci (Hons) – FY1 doctor, Northern General Hospital, Sheffield, UK

Andrew Viggars MBChB (Hons) BMedSci (Hons) – FY1 doctor, Sheffield Children's Hospital, Sheffield, UK

Advisors:

L. Wyld BMedSci MBChB (Hons) PhD FRCS(Gen Surg) – Senior Lecturer in Surgical Oncology and Honorary Consultant Surgeon. Academic Unit of Surgical Oncology, University of Sheffield, Royal Hallamshire Hospital, Sheffield, UK

J.P. Garner MBChB MD MRCS(Glasg) FRCS FRCSEd(Gen Surg) – Consultant General & Colorectal Surgeon, Rotherham NHS Foundation Trust, Rotherham and Defense Medical Services, Rothertham, UK

D.J. Rosario MBChB MD FRCS(Urol) – Senior Lecturer in Oncology and Hon. Consultant in Urology. Sheffield Teaching Hospitals NHS Trust, Royal Hallamshire Hospital, Sheffield, UK

A. Nassef MBBCh MSc MD FRCSEd FRCSEd(Gen Surg) – Consultant Vascular Surgeon. Sheffield Teaching Hospitals NHS Trust, Northern General Hospital, Sheffield, UK

A. Hormis MBChB FCARCSI AFICM – Consultant in Anaesthesia and Intensive Care Medicine, Rotherham NHS Foundation Trust, Rotherham, UK

EDITOR-IN-CHIEF:

Rory MacKinnon MBChB BSc(Hons) – GP Trainee Year 2, Crawcrook Medical Centre, Crawcrook, Tyne and Wear, UK

SERIES EDITORS:

Sally Keat BMedSci MBChB – Formally FY2 doctor, Chesterfield Royal Hospital, Chesterfield, UK

Thomas Locke BSc MBChB – Formally FY2 doctor, Sheffield Teaching Hospitals, Sheffield, UK

Andrew Walker BMedSci MBChB – MRCP (London), BHF Clinical Research Fellow and Honorary Specialist Registrar in Cardiology, Leeds Teaching Hospitals NHS Trust, UK

Acknowledgements

The authors would like to thank Sue Pridham, Colorectal & Stoma Nurse Specialist, Northern Lincolnshire and Goole Hospitals NHS Trust, Scunthorpe General Hospital, Scunthorpe, UK, for her contribution towards the production of this book.

List of abbreviations

- (5-ASA) 5-Aminosalicylic acid
- (AAA) Abdominal aortic aneurysm
- (ABCDE) Airway, Breathing, Circulation, Disability, Environment
- (ABG) Arterial blood gas
- (ABPI) Ankle-brachial pressure index
- (ACE) Angiotensin converting enzyme
- (ACTH) Adrenocorticotropic hormone
- (ADH) Anti-diuretic hormone
- (ALI) Acute limb ischaemia
- (ALP) Alkaline phosphatase
- (ALT) Alanine transaminase
- (APC) Adenomatous polyposis coli
- (ASA) American Society of Anesthesiologists
- (AST) Aspartate transaminase
- (BD) *bis in die* = twice in a day
- (BM) Boehringer–Mannheim = blood glucose test
- (BPH) Benign prostatic hypertrophy
- (CABG) Coronary artery bypass grafts
- (Ch.) Charière
- (CMV) Cytomegalovirus
- (COCP) Combined oral contraceptive pill
- (CPAP) Continuous positive airway pressure
- (Cr) Creatinine
- (CRC) Colorectal cancer
- (CRP) C-reactive protein
- (CSF) Cerebrospinal fluid
- (CVP) Central venous pressure
- (DCIS) Ductal carcinoma in situ
- (DM) Diabetes mellitus
- (DNA) Deoxyribonucleic acid
- (DPP) Dipeptidyl peptidase
- (D&V) Diahrrhoea and vomiting
- (EBV) Epstein–Barr virus
- (eGFR) Estimated glomerular filtration rate
- (EMD) Electromechanical dissociation
- (ER) Oestrogen receptor
- (ESR) Erythrocyte sedimentation rate
- (EVAR) Endovascular aneurysm repair/endovascular aortic repair
- (EVLA) Endovenous laser ablation

- (FBC) Full blood count
- (FNAC) Fine needle aspiration and cytology
- (Fr.) French
- (GGT) Gamma-glutamyltransferase
- (GLP) Glucagon-like peptide
- (HAV) Hepatitis A virus
- (Hb) Haemoglobin
- (HBV) Hepatitis B virus
- (HER2) Epidermal growth factor receptor (type 2)
- (HIV) Human immunodeficiency virus
- (HNPCC) Hereditary non-polyposis colorectal cancer
- (HR) Heart rate
- (HRT) Hormone replacement therapy
- (ICA) Internal carotid artery
- (ICU) Intensive care unit
- (I&D) Incision and drainage
- (IHD) Ischaemic heart disease
- (IM) Intramuscular
- (INR) International normalised ratio
- (IV) Intravenous
- (IVC) Inferior vena cava
- (JVP) Jugular venous pressure
- (K) Potassium
- (KUB) Kidney, ureters, bladder
- (LA) Local anaesthetic
- (LDH) Lactate dehydrogenase
- (LIF) Left iliac fossa
- (LRTI) Lower respiratory tract infection
- (LUQ) Left upper quadrant
- (LV) Left ventricle
- (MC&S) Microscopy, culture & sensitivity
- (MCV) Mean cell volume
- (MDT) Multidisciplinary team
- (MEN) Multiple endocrine neoplasia
- (MMG) Mammogram
- (MRA) Magnetic resonance angiography
- (MRI) Magnetic resonance imaging
- (MSU) Mid-stream urine
- (Na) Sodium
- (NBM) Nil by mouth
- (NCEPOD) National Confidential Enquiry into Patient Outcomes and Deaths
- (NHS) National Health Service

- (NICE) National Institute of Clinical Excellence
- (OD) *Omne in die* = once daily
- (OGD) Oesophagogastroduodenoscopy
- (PEC) Percutaneous endoscopic colostomy
- (PEG) Percutaneous endoscopic gastrostomy
- (PMH) Past medical history
- (PO) Per oral
- (PONV) Post-operative nausea & vomiting
- (PR) Per rectum
- (PT) Prothrombin time
- (PUJ) Pelviureteric junction
- (RIF) Right iliac fossa
- (RR) Respiratory rate
- (SBA) Single best answer
- (SC) Subcutaneous
- (SFJ) Sapheno–femoral junction
- (SLE) Systemic lupus erythematosis
- (SPJ) Sapheno–popliteal junction
- (STI) Sexually transmitted infection
- (T3) Tri-iodothyronine
- (T4) Thyroxine
- (TB) Tuberculosis
- (TIA) Transient ischaemic attack
- (TRAM) Transverse rectus abdominis myocutaneous (flap)
- (TSH) Thyroid stimulating hormone
- (U&Es) Urea and electrolytes
- (UGI) Upper gastrointestinal
- (UV) Ultraviolet
- (VTE) Venous thrombolism

An explanation of the text

The book is divided into two parts: general surgery revision notes and
a self-assessment section. We have used bullet points to keep the text concise
and supplemented this with a range of diagrams, pictures and MICRO-boxes
(explained below).

Where possible we have endeavoured to include treatment options for each
condition. Nevertheless, drug sensitivities and clinical practices are constantly
under review, so always check your local guidelines for up-to-date information.

MICRO-facts

These boxes expand on the text and contain clinically relevant facts and
memorable summaries of the essential information.

MICRO-print

These boxes contain additional information to the text that may interest
certain readers but is not essential for everybody to learn.

MICRO-case

These boxes contain clinical cases relevant to the text and include a
number of summary bullet points to highlight the key learning
objectives.

MICRO-reference

These boxes contain references to important clinical research and
national guidance.

Part I

General surgery

1 Pre-operative care

1.1 PRE-OPERATIVE ASSESSMENT IN THE ELECTIVE PATIENT

- The aim of pre-operative assessment is to maximise patient safety and minimise the complications of surgery by identifying potential problems and optimising patients before surgery.
- The extent of pre-operative preparation depends on several factors, mainly:
    - the timing of surgery (i.e. how urgent it is);
    - the nature of surgery (i.e. minor or major procedure);
    - the patient's past medical history and current status.

MICRO-facts

The National Confidential Enquiry into Patient Outcome and Deaths (NCEPOD) defines the timing of operations as follows:
- elective (planned procedures);
- scheduled (early surgery, e.g. within 2 weeks for malignancy);
- urgent (as soon as possible after resuscitation and within 24 hours);
- emergency (life-saving procedure with resuscitation alongside surgery).

MICRO-print

American Society of Anesthesiologists (ASA) grading:
- 1 = Healthy individual with no systemic disease.
- 2 = Mild systemic disease, not limiting activity.
- 3 = Severe systemic disease that limits activity but is not incapacitating.
- 4 = Incapacitating systemic disease which is constantly life-threatening.
- 5 = A moribund patient who is not expected to live 24 hours with or without surgery.

1.1.1 HISTORY AND EXAMINATION

- All patients should have a thorough history taken. Many units now have specially designed forms to ensure all areas are adequately explored. It is important to remember that the junior doctor who undertakes the pre-operative assessment may be the only person to take a detailed history and will often uncover important factors regarding the patient's peri-operative care.
- It is important that if such a critical factor is identified or an abnormal result is found, it is communicated to the consultants team before surgery, as this may avoid preventable complications or cancellation of the operation.
  - For example, identification that a patient is on clopidogrel, which must be stopped before elective surgery to reduce the risk of haemorrhage, or identification of undiagnosed aortic stenosis.
- Pre-operative assessment is therefore a very responsible role.
- A detailed, systematic history covering all areas is required.

History of presenting complaint

- Check that the condition has not worsened since the patient was listed, which may need to be communicated back to the surgeon.

> **MICRO-case**
>
> As the doctor in a pre-assessment clinic you see a man with oesophageal cancer who is due to undergo surgery. He is anaemic and appears emaciated. You discuss this with the consultant, who requests that the patient be admitted for pre-operative blood transfusion and nutritional support.

Past medical history

- In particular focussing on cardiovascular disease (including hypertension), respiratory disease, renal disease, diabetes and significant obesity.
- If a disease is identified, it should be optimally managed pre-operatively, so it is not enough to simply document 'hypertension'.
  - The level of control should be checked and if sub-optimal, steps taken to improve it. This may necessitate liaison with the GP or hospital specialist responsible for the care of this illness and delaying the planned surgery by contacting the consultant's team.

Drug history

- Particular care is needed to ensure this is accurate with correct drug names, doses and administration times. If necessary, contact the GP for verification.
- Certain drugs should be flagged up to the consultant's team, as they may have a significant impact on the surgery. These include:

- anticoagulants (see Section 1.3.6);
- steroids (see Section 1.3.9);
- anti-diabetic medication (see Section 1.3.10);
- chemotherapeutic agents: blood counts need to be carefully monitored;
- ACE-inhibitors (e.g. ramipril) and angiotensin II receptor antagonists (e.g. losartan), which should be omitted on the morning of surgery.
- The following medications should **not** be stopped prior to surgery:
  - antihypertensives, especially beta-blockers (e.g. atenolol);
  - other cardiac medications (e.g. digoxin);
  - inhalers, especially steroid inhalers (e.g. beclomethasone);
  - analgesics;
  - proton pump inhibitors (PPIs) (e.g. omeprazole).

Allergies

- These should be documented and described in terms of severity.
- In latex allergy the surgical team should be informed, as these patients should be first on the operating list and may require special equipment.

Social history

- Important issues include:
  - Jehovah's Witnesses who refuse blood products;
  - patients who have inadequate support on discharge where timely input from social services may ensure smooth discharge planning;
  - smoking and illicit substance abuse.

Family history

- A family history of cardiovascular disease or hyperlipidaemia may trigger more detailed assessments.

Systematic enquiry

- All domains should be explored: cardiovascular, respiratory, gastrointestinal, renal, musculoskeletal, and neurological systems.

Exercise tolerance

- Should be documented and if poor, further investigation instigated.

Previous anaesthetic problems

- Previous reactions, airway problems or post-operative nausea or vomiting should be noted.

Examination

- A full physical examination is required for all patients.

1.1.2 RELEVANT INVESTIGATIONS

- Not all investigations are necessary for all patients. Assess the age and comorbidities of the patient, as well as the type of procedure planned (Table 1.1).

Table 1.1 Indications for pre-operative investigations in elective patients.

PRE-OPERATIVE TEST	INDICATIONS FOR USE IN ELECTIVE PATIENTS
Full blood count (FBC)	All patients undergoing major surgery. All patients with cardiovascular or renal disease. Consider in all patients with ASA grade 2 or more.
Urea and electrolytes (U&E)	All patients undergoing major surgery. All patients with renal or cardiovascular disease. All patients over 60 years with ASA grade 2 or more.
Liver function tests (LFTs)	All patients with a history of liver disease, jaundice, alcohol excess, intravenous drug use. All patients with abnormal nutritional state or metabolic disease. All patients taking hepatotoxic drugs.
Blood glucose	All diabetic patients undergoing surgery. All patients with renal disease or if glycosuria or ketonuria are present on urinalysis. Consider in all patients aged over 60 years or the obese.
Clotting screen	All patients with a past medical history or family history of bleeding or clotting disorders and those with known liver disease. All patients taking anticoagulants. All patients undergoing major surgery.
Group and save cross-match	All patients undergoing intermediate, major, major-plus or laparoscopic surgery should be grouped and saved. In procedures where there is significant anticipated blood loss, e.g. abdominal aortic aneurysm (AAA) repair, patients should be cross-matched. All patients with coagulopathies or anaemia.
12-Lead electrocardiography (ECG)	All patients with cardiovascular disease or diabetes. Consider in all patients over 40 years of age, especially if there are cardiovascular risk factors (e.g. smoking, hypertension) or when undergoing major surgery.

Table 1.1 (*Continued*)

PRE-OPERATIVE TEST	INDICATIONS FOR USE IN ELECTIVE PATIENTS
Chest x-ray (CXR)	All patients over 60 years of age should have had a CXR within the preceding 12 months. All patients with cardiorespiratory disease, malignancy, thyroid goitre or those undergoing thoracic surgery.

MICRO-print

NICE grades of elective surgery:

1. (Minor): e.g. excision of skin lesion, drainage of breast abscess.
2. (Intermediate): e.g. inguinal hernia repair, varicose vein stripping.
3. (Major): e.g. thyroidectomy.
4. (Major plus): e.g. colonic resection, thoracic procedures.

1.1.3 SPECIFIC INVESTIGATIONS

- The following are not routinely required but may be required in certain patients (Table 1.2).

Table 1.2 Indications for specific pre-operative investigations in elective patients.

PRE-OPERATIVE TEST	INDICATIONS FOR USE IN ELECTIVE PATIENTS
Sickle cell test	Consider in African or Caribbean patients undergoing surgery. All patients with a family history of sickle cell disease.
Echocardiography	All patients with significant cardiovascular disease undergoing major surgery. All patients diagnosed with a new murmur.
Pulmonary function tests (PFTs)	All patients with significant respiratory disease undergoing major surgery.

MICRO-reference

NICE guidelines: Clinical guideline 3: Preoperative tests—The use of routine preoperative tests for elective surgery. http://www.nice.org.uk/nicemedia/live/10920/29090/29090.pdf

General surgery

1.2 PRE-OPERATIVE ASSESSMENT IN THE EMERGENCY SURGICAL PATIENT

- In the emergency setting, preparation for theatre is about optimisation to give the patient the best possible chance of a good surgical outcome.
- In patients with severe comorbidity, NCEPOD recommends:
  - communication between surgeon and anaesthetist pre-operatively;
  - adequate pre-operative investigation;
  - appropriate grade of surgeon (minimising operating time and blood loss);
  - adequate resuscitation;
  - availability of critical care bed.
- It should not be forgotten that emergency admissions may require urgent surgery, and so a thorough history and examination should be performed by the admitting doctor, as described above (Section 1.1.1).

1.2.1 PRE-OPERATIVE INVESTIGATIONS IN EMERGENCY PATIENTS

- All emergency general surgical patients should have an appropriate set of blood test results available prior to surgery, including FBC, U&E, LFTs, glucose, clotting screen, group and save or cross-match depending on the type of surgery, their comorbid conditions and the underlying acute illness.
- All sexually active women of child-bearing age should have a pregnancy test.
- Patients admitted with an acute abdomen, where perforation of a viscus is part of the differential diagnosis, should have an erect chest x-ray.
- Any patients with tachycardia and all adults aged 40 over years should have a baseline ECG, as should anyone with a cardiac, hypertensive or respiratory history.
- All patients should have a simple urinalysis.
- An ABG may be relevant in patients with significant respiratory disease and those with acute sepsis, pancreatitis or suspected intestinal ischaemia where a metabolic acidosis may develop.

1.3 HOW TO MANAGE CONDITIONS OF SPECIAL RELEVANCE

1.3.1 RECENT MYOCARDIAL INFARCTION (MI)

- Avoid elective surgery [unless urgent or coronary artery bypass grafting (CABG)] for >6 months as risk of re-infarction is elevated.
- Specific relevant investigations:
  - up-to-date ECG and echocardiogram.

General surgery

- Continue all normal cardiovascular medications.
- Consider stopping anti-platelets 10 days prior to surgery.

1.3.2 AORTIC STENOSIS (AS)

- Patients with severe AS should not undergo elective surgery without prior consideration of valvular replacement.
- Specific relevant investigations:
  - echo to assess the pressure gradient across the valve and its area—the normal gradient is only a few mmHg.
- Prophylactic antibiotics may be required, although the indications for this have recently been substantially reduced.
  - See NICE guidelines for criteria and type (see micro-reference box).
- Patients may be on anticoagulants.
- Avoid tachycardia and hypotension as patients are at risk of MI.
  - Diastolic filling is reduced due to left ventricular hypertrophy.

MICRO-facts

LV-aortic gradient:
- Mild: <20mmHg.
- Moderate: 20–50mmHg.
- Severe: >50mmHg.

MICRO-facts

Aortic valve reduction area:
- Normal: 2.6–3.5 cm².
- Mild: 1.6–2.5 cm².
- Moderate: 1.0–1.5 cm².
- Severe: <1.0 cm².

MICRO-reference

NICE clinical guideline 64: Prophylaxis against infective endocarditis: Antimicrobial prophylaxis against infective endocarditis in adults and children undergoing interventional procedures. http://www.nice.org.uk/nicemedia/live/10920/29090/29090.pdf

1.3.3 ATRIAL FIBRILLATION (AF)

- Can precipitate cardiac failure if inadequately rate-controlled peri-operatively.
- Discuss management plan with anaesthetist.
- May be on warfarin (see Section 1.3.6).

General surgery

- Specific relevant investigations:
  - ECG to assess rate and rhythm (if paroxysmal);
  - INR if on warfarin.

1.3.4 CARDIAC FAILURE

- Postpone surgery until stable and optimised on medication.
- Important to carefully control fluid balance to avoid overload.
- Specific relevant investigations:
  - U&Es as diuretics and ACE-inhibitors can cause renal impairment.
  - CXR to assess for disease severity and fluid overload.
  - ECG and echocardiogram to assess LV function.

1.3.5 PACEMAKERS

- Check the reason for insertion of the pacemaker (usually bradyarrhythmias).
- Check the type of pacemaker.
  - Implantable cardioverter defibrillators (ICDs) should be turned off prior to surgery and turned back on in recovery.
- Specific relevant investigations:
  - An ECG to demonstrate normal function of the pacemaker.
- A recent pacemaker check is essential to confirm battery life and normal function.

> **MICRO-print**
> Bipolar diathermy is safest in patients with pacemakers and monopolar should be avoided.

1.3.6 PATIENTS TAKING ANTICOAGULANTS

- If on warfarin, it is important to weigh the risk of stopping the medication against the risk of bleeding intra-operatively, and this risk varies with the indication for therapy.
  - Patients on warfarin for AF, for example, are not at great risk if they stop taking it and so may simply omit the drug for 5–7 days pre-operatively.
  - Patients on warfarin for metallic heart valves, however, are at high risk of thromboembolism if the INR is normalised and so should have cover with low molecular weight heparin (LMWH) or IV heparin.
- In the emergency setting, reversal of warfarin may be required quickly and so drugs such as vitamin K, fresh frozen plasma (FFP) or prothrombin complex concentrate may be used.
  - This requires discussion with haematology for advice on appropriate product and dosage.

General surgery

- Anti-platelet medications should be omitted pre-operatively.
  - Stop clopidogrel 7–10 days pre-operatively.
  - Stop dipyridamole 7 days pre-operatively.
  - Omit aspirin on the day of surgery.
- For patients on anticoagulants, please consult your local guidelines.

1.3.7 RECENT CEREBROVASCULAR ACCIDENT (CVA)

- Avoid elective surgery (unless urgent or carotid endarterectomy) for >6 weeks.
  - This is because autoregulation of cerebral blood pressure is disrupted following a CVA, and normal ability to cope with fluctuations of cerebral blood pressure caused by anaesthetic agents is impaired. This increases the risk of a further peri-operative CVA.

1.3.8 HYPERTHYROIDISM

- Patients with hyperthyroidism are at risk of thyrotoxic crisis, AF and bleeding.
- Efforts should be made to make the patient euthyroid prior to surgery.
- Specific relevant investigations:
  - Thyroid function tests (TFTs), ECG, CXR.
- AF may resolve on treating the underlying thyroid disease, but patients may require rate control with beta-blockers, digoxin, verapamil or amiodarone.
- Anti-thyroid drugs may increase bleeding in thyroid surgery, and are often stopped 10–14 days prior to surgery.

MICRO-facts

Check for a large goitre and tracheal deviation in hyperthyroid patients, as this can impact on airway management.

1.3.9 IMMUNOSUPPRESSION

- Surgical patients on long-term steroid therapy are at risk of Addisonian crisis.
  - These should be continued throughout surgery, as their use results in adrenal suppression leading to an impaired stress response.
- Patients unable to take their oral steroids will require IV hydrocortisone.
- If patients are taking <10 mg of prednisolone daily (or equivalent dose of other steroid), they need no additional steroid cover.
- If taking >10 mg daily, patients will need 25 mg IV hydrocortisone at induction of anaesthesia and additional cover post-op dependent on the type of surgery.

General surgery

1.3.10 DIABETES MELLITUS

- Diabetic patients who undergo surgery are at risk of multiple complications (see Figure 1.1).
- Ensure the patient is first on the operating list to optimise glycaemic control.
- Specific relevant investigations:
  - U&E, blood glucose, ECG.
- Adjust medication according to the timing and extent of surgery and in consultation with the anaesthetist (see Table 1.3).
- Patients may require a variable rate insulin infusion (VRII), particularly if starved for a substantial period or if they have decompensated diabetes (e.g. in the presence of sepsis).
- BMs should be monitored regularly to ensure good control.

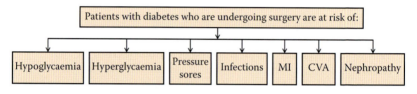

Figure 1.1 Specific risks in diabetic surgical patients.

Table 1.3 Alterations in diabetic medication before surgery taken from NHS diabetes summary (see micro-reference).

DRUG	PATIENT FOR A.M. SURGERY	PATIENT FOR P.M. SURGERY
Insulin OD	No change to dose.	No change to dose.
Insulin BD	½ a.m. dose, normal p.m. dose.	½ a.m. dose, normal p.m. dose.
Insulin BD separate short and intermediate agents	½ **total** a.m. dose as intermediate-acting insulin, normal p.m. dose.	½ **total** a.m. dose as intermediate-acting insulin, normal p.m. dose.
Insulin 3, 4 or 5 injections daily	Basal bolus regimens: Omit a.m. and lunchtime short-acting insulin keeping basal dose normal. Premixed a.m. regimens: ½ a.m. dose and omit lunchtime dose.	Normal a.m. dose, omit lunchtime dose.
Acarbose or meglitinide (e.g. repalinide)	Omit a.m. dose if NBM.	Give a.m. dose if eating.

General surgery

Table 1.3 (*Continued*)

DRUG	PATIENT FOR A.M. SURGERY	PATIENT FOR P.M. SURGERY
Sulphonylurea (e.g. gliclazide)	Omit a.m. dose.	Omit a.m. dose if OD, omit a.m. and p.m. dose if BD.
Pioglitazone or metformin	Normal dosing.	Normal dosing.
DPP IV inhibitor (e.g. sitagliptin) or GLP-analogue (e.g. exenatide)	Omit on day of surgery.	Omit on day of surgery.

MICRO-reference

Management of adults with diabetes undergoing surgery and elective procedures: Improving standards. NHS diabetes summary (April 2011). http://www.diabetes.nhs.uk/document.php?o=225

1.3.11 MORBID OBESITY

- Operations are made more complicated due to:
  - Harder to manually handle larger patients.
- Special equipment may be required, such as larger operating tables, beds and special hoists. Not every hospital will have these.
- Increased prevalence of comorbidities, e.g. IHD, DM, gallstones, etc.
- Poor airway for anaesthetic intubation.
- Obesity may predispose to multiple complications (see Figure 1.2).
- Specific relevant investigations:
  - ECG, blood glucose, respiratory function tests, including spirometry, ABG and CXR.

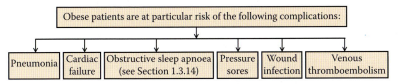

Figure 1.2 Complications specific to obese patients undergoing surgery.

1.3.12 RENAL FAILURE

- Manage all renal failure patients jointly with a nephrologist.
- Mild chronic renal failure is common in the elderly surgical patient.

General surgery

- Delay elective surgery to allow optimisation and stabilisation of the condition.
- Avoid nephrotoxic drugs, e.g. gentamicin.
- Make sure hydration is maintained pre-operatively.
- Severe renal failure.
  - Risk of fluid overload, electrolyte imbalances, metabolic acidosis and anaemia of renal failure.
  - Uraemia is immunosuppressant so ensure prophylactic antibiotics.
- Monitor urine output, plasma electrolytes, creatinine, urea and bicarbonate.
  - Check potassium regularly, as having a general anaesthetic (GA) increases the risk of hyperkalaemia.
- Haemodialysis patients should have dialysis more than 24 hours pre-operatively to allow the effects of heparin to wear off.
- Patients using peritoneal dialysis having abdominal surgery may need to be converted to haemodialysis pre- and post-operatively.

1.3.13 COPD

- Lung function decreases with the use of GA, so alternatives, such as regional anaesthesia, may be considered.
- Optimise medical therapy with nebulisers, oxygen and steroids as required.
- Advise smoking cessation 4–8 weeks prior to surgery.
- Use of chest physiotherapy at least twice a day:
  - passive, e.g. breathing exercises;
  - active, e.g. postural drainage.
- May need to book a bed on HDU for post-operative non-invasive ventilation.
- Specific relevant investigations:
  - Assess lung function using spirometry, ABG and CXR.

1.3.14 OBSTRUCTIVE SLEEP APNOEA

- As with chronic obstructive pulmonary disease (COPD), consider alternatives to GA.
- Be cautious with use of sedatives and opiates, as these agents can decrease respiratory function and increase the frequency of apnoeic episodes.
- If patient is currently using CPAP, he or she will require this post-operatively.
- May require a bed on the high-dependency unit (HDU) post-operatively.
- Specific relevant investigations:
  - Assess lung function using spirometry, ABG and CXR.

1.3.15 LIVER DISEASE

Patients with liver disease are at risk of several complications (see Figure 1.3).

- Patients with liver disease may be classified using the Child–Pugh criteria (Table 1.4).

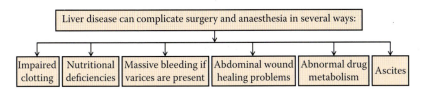

Figure 1.3 Complications specific to patients with liver disease undergoing surgery.

Table 1.4 Components of the Child–Pugh scoring system for liver disease.

SCORE	1 POINT	2 POINTS	3 POINTS
Bilirubin	<34 µmol/L	34–50 µmol/L	>50 µmol/L
Albumin	>35 g/L	28–35 g/L	<28 g/L
INR	<1.7	1.7–2.3	>2.3
Ascites	None	Mild	Moderate–severe
Encephalopathy	None	Grade I or II	Grade III or IV

- Surgical risks vary with the score, and in those with a high score all but the most critical, life-saving surgery are contraindicated.
- Specific relevant investigations:
    - FBC, clotting screen, U&E, LFT and bone profile.
- Patients should have close monitoring of blood sugar, as they have defective glycolysis and gluconeogenesis.
- Patients with deranged clotting may need vitamin K pre-operatively for several days or require fresh frozen plasma (FFP) peri-operatively.
- Prophylactic antibiotics are indicated.

1.3.16 INFECTION

- Any patient with a transmissible infection should be placed last on the operating list to avoid the risk of infecting other patients.
    - Universal precautions should be strictly adhered to (see protection of the surgeon, Section 1.5.3) in patients with category III infections (e.g. HIV, Hepatitis, TB).
- Surgery should be delayed if possible in any patient with an acute respiratory or urinary tract infection.
- Infection at the surgical site can pose problems, including:
    - Poor wound healing.
        - Actively infected wounds may be left open to encourage healing by secondary intent.
        - Drains may be used to drain local infection where appropriate.
    - Local anaesthetic may be ineffective due to the acidic local microenvironment caused by sepsis.

General surgery

1.4 PREPARATION FOR THEATRE

1.4.1 FASTING

- Patients should be fasted pre-operatively if having a general or regional anaesthesia:
    - May take food or drinks containing milk up to 6 hours before.
    - May take clear fluids up to 2 hours before.
- If fasted for a substantial period, patients will require an intravenous infusion (IVI) of fluids.
    - Note that elective patients will not require IVI, as they can drink up to 2 hours before surgery.
    - Ensure an appropriate gauge IV cannula is inserted in an appropriate location (e.g. the back of the non-dominant hand).

1.4.2 MEDICATIONS

- It is important to take a thorough drug history and ensure the appropriate medications are prescribed for the patient's hospital stay.
- All surgical patients should be assessed for venous thromboembolic prophylaxis (see Section 1.4.3).
- Ensure 'special' medications are prescribed (see local guidelines), e.g.:
    - bowel preparation or enemas for colonic and rectal procedures;
    - antibiotic prophylaxis.

1.4.3 THROMBOPROPHYLAXIS

- Appropriate thromboprophylaxis (Table 1.5) should be chosen according to risk (see Figure 1.4).
- LMWH should be given early the evening before (e.g. 1800 h) major surgery (i.e. >12 hours before spinals) and should be prescribed post-operatively.
- The presence of foot pulses should be confirmed before prescribing stockings.

> **MICRO-reference**
> NICE (2010). *Venous thromboembolism: Reducing the risk* [CG92]. London: National Institute for Health and Clinical Excellence. http://www.nice.org.uk/nicemedia/live/12695/47197/47197.pdf

Table 1.5 Types of thromboprophylaxis.

MEDICAL PROPHYLAXIS	PHARMACOLOGICAL PROPHYLAXIS
Anti-embolic stockings	Fondaparinux
Foot impulse devices	LMWH—usually Clexane 40 mg/24 h S/C
Intermittent pneumatic compression devices	Unfractionated heparin

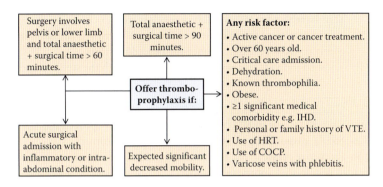

Figure 1.4 Patients who require thromboprophylaxis.

1.4.4 DOCUMENTATION

- Patients should all have an admission clerking in the notes.
- Informed consent should have been taken and documented.
  - This should ideally be done by the operating surgeon or someone who is able to perform the surgery himself or herself. In all cases the person taking consent must be fully aware of the risks of the procedure and have had training in taking consent.
- The surgical site should be marked where appropriate (i.e. laterality should be confirmed—e.g. **left** breast mastectomy).
- All medications should be prescribed on the drug chart, which should be available to go with the patient to theatre.

1.5 FIRST TIME IN THE OPERATING THEATRE

1.5.1 THEATRE ETIQUETTE

- The dignity of patients should be maintained at all time.
- Appropriate clothing (e.g. theatre scrubs, hats, shoes and identification badges) should be worn at all times in theatre areas.
- Jewellery should be removed.
- A quiet environment should be maintained within theatre to allow effective communication between the members of the operating team.
- When working in theatres, individuals should ensure they have up-to-date hepatitis B vaccination.

1.5.2 STERILITY WHEN OPERATING OR ASSISTING

- You should be supervised and shown how to scrub correctly when attending theatre for the first time.
  - Once you are scrubbed and gowned up, you must not touch any non-sterile objects (e.g. rubbing your nose, adjusting your glasses or theatre mask are common mistakes made by first-time students).

General surgery

- Your hands and arms should be kept close to your chest (e.g. in a 'prayer' position) to avoid them becoming unsterilised and should be gently rested on the drapes once the procedure starts.
- Only scrubbed individuals should come in contact with the sterile drapes.

1.5.3 PROTECTION OF THE SURGEON

- Universal precautions should be ensured during invasive procedures.
  - Sterile, disposable gloves and gowns should be worn.
  - Protective eyewear and face masks should also be worn.
- Treat all needle-stick injuries seriously.
  - Hepatitis B carries a 25% transmission rate following needle-stick.
  - Hepatitis C has no vaccine and carries a 2% transmission rate. There is no post-exposure prophylaxis for hepatitis C.
    - Management of exposure includes early identification of infection and specialist referral.
  - In the case of a needle-stick injury in a known HIV-positive patient, post-exposure prophylaxis should be given within 24 hours.
    - Anti-retroviral drugs should be prescribed to maintain a low viral load and reduce the risk of transmission.

MICRO-facts

In case of a needle-stick injury:
- First-aid treatment:
  - If the mouth or eyes are involved, they should be washed thoroughly with sterile water.
  - If skin is punctured, bleeding should be encouraged and the wound washed with water and with soap or chlorhexidine.
    - It should not be scrubbed or sucked.
- Immediate action:
  - A blood sample from the exposed person should be taken and the incident should be reported to Occupational Health.
  - The patient should be informed of the incident and consent should be gained for a blood sample to test for transmissible infections.
- Follow-up should occur with Occupational Health to ensure there has been no transmission of blood-borne infections.

MICRO-reference

NHS employers document on needlestick injuries (2012). http://www.nhsemployers.org/Aboutus/Publications/Documents/Needlestick%20injury.pdf

1.6 INCISIONS

- Surgical incisions may tell you a significant amount of information about a patient's post-surgical history.

1.6.1 PRACTICAL CONSIDERATIONS

- There are several elements that should be considered when choosing an appropriate surgical incision:
  - **Access:** It should be placed to provide appropriate access to the required organs and be large enough to work in.
  - **Orientation:** Incisions should ideally be placed along Langer's lines (lines of skin tension) or in skin creases to aid healing and reduce distortion and scarring.
  - **Underlying anatomy:** Incisions should be placed to avoid damaging important underlying structures (e.g. nerves and blood vessels).
  - Good cosmesis.

1.6.2 ABDOMINAL INCISIONS

- Common abdominal incisions are shown in Figure 1.5.
  - Rooftop incision.
    - Also known as double Kocher's.
    - Good access to liver and spleen.
    - Used for radical pancreatic and gastric surgery.
  - Kocher's incision.
    - Situated 3 cm below and parallel to the costal margin.
    - Used for open cholecystectomy (on the right) or splenectomy (on the left).
  - Midline laparotomy.
    - Through the linea alba.
    - Good access to most abdominal structures.

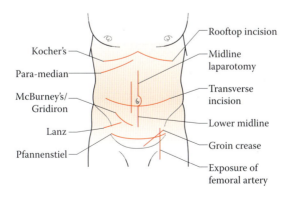

Figure 1.5 Common abdominal incisions. (From: Self-drawn.)

General surgery

- – Commonly used for open colorectal, gastric, aortic and trauma surgery.
- Para-median.
  - – Historic, now rarely used. Has been replaced by midline laparotomy.
- Transverse incision.
  - – Less painful than midline laparotomy.
  - – Used as an alternative for open colorectal and aortic surgery.
- McBurney's/gridiron.
  - – Centred on McBurney's point.
  - – Used for appendicectomy.
- Lanz.
  - – Lower than McBurney's incision. Better cosmetic result (may be hidden by bikini line).
  - – Used for appendicectomy.
- Groin crease.
  - – 1–2 cm above and parallel to the inguinal ligament.
  - – Used for open inguinal hernia repairs.
- Pfannenstiel.
  - – Commonly used in gynaecological surgery, e.g. caesarean section.

2 Lumps and bumps

2.1 ABDOMINAL WALL HERNIAE

- A hernia is the protrusion of a viscus, or part of a viscus, through an opening in the cavity that normally holds it in place.
- Patients with hernias are at risk of developing the complications associated with these conditions.
- They are common presentations to general surgeons and often come up in exams (see Figure 2.1—the sites of common herniae).

2.1.1 AETIOLOGY

- Congenital, e.g. umbilical.
- Acquired.
  - Weakness in the abdominal wall muscles (rectus sheath, external oblique, internal oblique, transversus abdominis).
  - Raised intra-abdominal pressure, e.g.:
    - heavy lifting;
    - straining (valsalva manoeuvre);
    - coughing;
    - free fluid (ascites);
    - obesity;
    - pregnancy.
  - Iatrogenic, i.e. weakened abdominal wall after surgery (incisional herniae).

2.1.2 CLINICAL FEATURES

- New lump, which may be reducible (i.e. can be pushed back in with gentle pressure).
- Aching or dragging sensation at the site.
- 'Tearing' sensation at formation on lifting, straining or coughing.
- Acute pain and tenderness may indicate strangulation.
- May present with features of bowel obstruction (see Section 6.12).

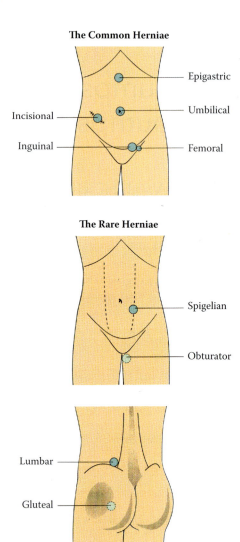

Figure 2.1 The sites of herniae. (From: *Browse's Introduction to the Symptoms and Signs of Surgical Disease*, 4th Edition, Figure 14.1.)

2.1.3 COMPLICATIONS

Incarceration

- Hernia is irreducible due to a small neck or adhesions. It is not usually painful. If pain or tenderness is present in an irreducible hernia, then think about strangulation (see following page).

Obstruction

- Pressure on the bowel at the hernia neck obstructs the bowel lumen, causing small bowel obstruction (most commonly).

Strangulation

- The blood supply to the hernia contents (e.g. bowel or omentum) is compromised due to pressure at the neck, which may lead to necrosis.

MICRO-facts

Abdominal wall herniae commonly contain omentum or small bowel, as these are the most mobile contents of the abdomen. However, other internal organs, such as the appendix (Amyand's hernia), large bowel, ovary or even bladder, may be contained within a hernia.

2.1.4 MANAGEMENT

- Surgical repair to prevent complications.
    - The hernia defect is exposed, the contents of the hernia replaced in the abdominal cavity, and the defect is either simply closed with sutures, or in some cases the repair is reinforced with plastic mesh.
    - Many repairs are now performed laparoscopically (e.g. inguinal hernias).
- Conservative management is sometimes appropriate in a wide-necked, asymptomatic hernia in a frail patient. A truss may be used to support the defect.
    - However local anaesthetic (LA) open repairs are generally safe and well tolerated with good results.

2.1.5 POST-OPERATIVE COMPLICATIONS

- Recurrence rates are low (2–3% in simple inguinal hernias), but may be higher in more complex hernias (e.g. up to 10% in primary incisional hernia repairs).
    - Patients should avoid heavy lifting for 6 weeks with a phased return to normal activity so as to avoid putting pressure on the repair.
- Surgical wound infection.
    - This may be further complicated by mesh infection, necessitating mesh removal.
- In inguinal hernia repairs there is a risk of testicular ischaemia or atrophy, presumed due to damage of the spermatic cord (and hence the testicular blood supply).
    - This risk is higher with recurrent repairs.

General surgery

MICRO-facts

In males, inguinal herniae often descend into the scrotum (due to the embryological pathway of the testes through the inguinal canal).

2.1.6 SPECIFIC TYPES

Inguinal hernia

- This is the most common type of abdominal wall hernia.
- Herniation occurs through the inguinal canal directly (through the back wall) or indirectly (through the deep inguinal ring) (see Figure 2.2).
- M:F ratio = 8:1 due to the fact that the hernia tract, the inguinal canal, is maintained patent by the presence of the testicular vessels on their way from the retroperitoneum to the scrotum.
- Indirect hernias descend through the deep inguinal ring (lateral to the inferior epigastric artery) through the canal and appear above and medial to the pubic tubercle.
  - If reduced, pressure over the deep ring should prevent re-herniation.
- Direct hernias push through the wall of the inguinal canal medial to the inferior epigastric artery and do not pass through the deep ring.
  - More common in the elderly when the muscles are weaker.

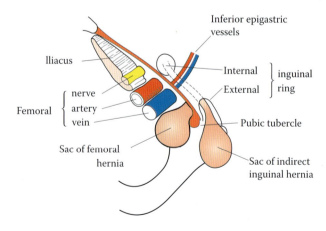

Figure 2.2 Anatomy of the inguinal canal and the relations of groin herniae. (From: *Bailey & Love's Short Practice of Surgery, 26th Edition*, Figure 57.4.)

Femoral

- Protrusion of abdominal contents into the femoral canal.
- F > M (but still less common than inguinal herniae in both sexes).
- Small swelling arising just below the inguinal ligament, lateral and inferior to the pubic tubercle.
- They are deeper and less mobile than other causes of lumps here.
- As the neck of the sac here is small, they are often irreducible, and 40–50% of femoral hernias are strangulated at presentation.

Epigastric

- These defects are often very small (0.5 cm).
- May only be herniation of extraperitoneal fat, although omentum or small bowel may also protrude.
- Weakness in the linea alba, anywhere between the xiphoid process and umbilicus.
- The hernia will be in the midline.
- There may be sharp pain at the site if extraperitoneal fat is trapped and infarcts.

Paraumbilical

- F > M.
- The defect is in the linea alba around the umbilicus.
- May contain omentum, transverse colon or small bowel.
- Often continue to grow in size and are likely to strangulate.
- They occur in the obese and females with poor muscle tone.

> **MICRO-print**
> Epigastric and paraumbilical herniae have an association with pregnancy as the rectus sheath muscles are stretched apart.

Umbilical

- Usually due to a congenital defect where the umbilical vessels emerge. Usually regress without intervention but occasionally need treatment.
  - May also present in adulthood.

Incisional

- Abdominal contents herniate through a defect created through an incision in the abdominal wall following abdominal surgery.
- Due to poor post-operative healing. Commonly secondary to wound infection, deep dehiscence, or excessive intra-abdominal pressure and lack of sufficient resting of the site after surgery.

General surgery

Spigelian

- Uncommon.
- Occur through the Spigelian fascia (formed by the internal oblique and transversus abdominis fascias) between fibres of external oblique.
- Protrude lateral to the rectus sheath.

MICRO-case

An elderly lady is admitted with nausea and vomiting. She has not opened her bowels for a day and is complaining of colicky abdominal pain. She is tachypnoeic and tachycardic, with a BP of 95/45 mmHg. On examination her abdomen is distended, but soft and non-tender. You commence fluid resuscitation and insert a urinary catheter. Her blood results are shown:

WCC	16.0×109/L.
Urea	12.3 mmol/L.
Creatinine	125 mmol/L.
ABG	Metabolic acidosis with a raised lactate.

You expose her from 'nipple to knees' and inspection of her groin reveals a 3-cm mass that is exquisitely tender, irreducible and the overlying skin appears dusky. She has a strangulated femoral hernia, and undergoes emergency repair of the hernia with resection of the necrotic small bowel.

Learning points:

- Hernias may present with obstruction or strangulation.
- When performing abdominal examination, fully expose the patient.
- A strangulated hernia is an emergency, requiring prompt diagnosis and treatment with resuscitation, antibiotics and rapid operative intervention.

2.2 HOW TO EXAMINE FOR GROIN HERNIAE

- Any groin lump may be painful; therefore care must be taken during examination.
- Both the groin and scrotum (in males) must be examined to define the origin of the lump.

2.2.1 EXAMINATION SEQUENCE

- Introduce yourself and ask permission to examine.
- Ensure a chaperone is present.
- Clean your hands.
- Ask if the area to be examined is painful.
- Expose the patient between groin and knees.

- Examine the patient lying **and** standing.
  - Gravity may show a hernia that is not obvious when the patient lies down.
  - A groin lump that disappears as the patient lies down is quite likely to be an inguinal hernia.
- Test for a cough impulse:
  - Place you fingers over the lump and ask the patient to cough. Examine both sides simultaneously to compare and prevent the necessity for the patient to cough repeatedly.
- Test for reducibility in both lying and standing positions.
  - Most inguinal hernias are reducible unless they are long-standing.
  - In contrast, half of all femoral hernias will not be reducible at presentation.
- Differentiate a femoral hernia from inguinal by the relation of the hernia neck to the pubic tubercle.
  - Inguinal hernias arise above and medial to the tubercle.
  - Femoral hernias arise below the inguinal ligament, lateral to the pubic tubercle.
- For inguinal hernias, once reduced, apply pressure over the deep inguinal ring (at the mid-point of the inguinal ligament) and ask the patient to cough.
  - If an inguinal hernia reappears medial to your fingers, it is direct.
  - If your pressure prevents an inguinal hernia from reappearing, it is indirect.
  - Note: Determination of whether a hernia is direct or indirect is a very inexact science and even the experts get this wrong. Additionally, it makes little difference to the way the hernia is treated.
- Examine the scrotum.
  - Does the lump extend down into the scrotum?
  - Can you get above it? If you can, this means the swelling is arising from the scrotum.
  - Is the testis present in the scrotal sac? Occasionally a torted ectopic testicle may present as a 'strangulated hernia'. If the testicle is not in the scrotum, surgical exploration must be preceded by informed consent for orchidectomy.
- Auscultate the hernia to see if bowel sounds are present. This will indicate that the lump is a hernia and whether it contains bowel.

2.3 BENIGN SOFT TISSUE SWELLINGS

- Soft tissue masses are very common, and the majority are of benign aetiology by a factor of 100:1.
  - The most common types are lipomas and sebaceous cysts, which are usually fairly easy to differentiate.
  - Rarer benign pathologies include neurofibromas and haemangiomas.

General surgery

- It is important to identify the risk factors for a more serious pathology, such as a soft tissue cancer (sarcoma) or other malignant pathology, such as a soft tissue metastasis from a visceral or skin cancer. The key warning signs are:
  - size greater than 5 cm;
  - submuscular location;
  - rapid increase in size;
  - painful;
  - signs or symptoms of local invasion/infiltration.

2.3.1 LIPOMA

- A lipoma is a common benign tumour of fatty tissue.
- May occur at any age but most commonly in adults aged 30–50 years.
- F = M.

> **MICRO-print**
> Multiple tender lipomata on the trunk are the hallmark of Dercum's disease.

Clinical features

- Soft, lobulated, pseudo-fluctuant.
- Normal overlying skin.
- Slow growing.
- Can arise in any connective tissue but usually in the subcutaneous fat.

Treatment

- Conservative management if not symptomatic or marginal excision if the patient wishes.
- May rarely undergo malignant change.

2.3.2 SEBACEOUS CYST

- Also known as an epidermoid cyst or Wen.
- These are retention cysts formed by obstruction to the mouth of sebaceous glands.

Clinical features (see Figure 2.3)

- Not common in childhood.
- Common areas include the scalp, face, neck, back, scrotum and vulva.
- Spherical, soft or firm.
- Contain caseous sebaceous material.
- Punctum (dimple at site of attachment to skin due to its epidermal origin).

Complications

- Infection and abscess formation.
- Ulceration.

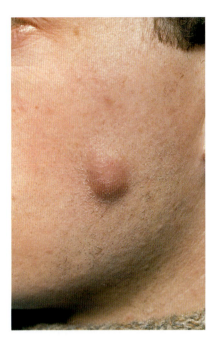

Figure 2.3 A small sebaceous cyst on the face. (From: *Browse's Introduction to the Symptoms and Signs of Surgical Disease, 4th Edition*, Figure 3.26.)

Treatment

- Excision under LA with an ellipse of skin to include the punctum.
- The entire sac must be removed; otherwise they are likely to reoccur.
- If infected, they require incision and drainage.

> **MICRO-print**
> Cock's peculiar tumour is an ulcerated sebaceous cyst that resembles a fungating carcinoma.

2.3.3 DERMOID CYST

- Congenital dermoid cyst.
    - Formed in utero when the skin dermatomes fuse.
    - Commonly found on the head and neck.
- Acquired (implantation) dermoids.
    - A piece of skin is implanted into the dermis as a result of trauma or surgery.
    - Common on the fingers.
- Investigation: Computed tomography (CT) scanning to exclude intracranial extension.
- Treatment: Simple excision.

General surgery

> **MICRO-print**
> When located at the outer end of the eyebrow, a congenital dermoid is known as external angular dermoid.

2.3.4 FIBROMA

- Fibromas are benign tumours arising from mesenchymal tissue.
- They are composed of fibrous connective tissue.

Clinical features

- They may be hard (many fibres and a few cells), e.g. keloid.
- They may be soft (many loosely connected cells, less fibres), e.g. skin tag.
- Can grow in all organs.

Treatment

- Excision if causing irritation.

2.3.5 NEUROFIBROMA

- These are benign tumours arising from the connective tissue element of peripheral nerves.

Clinical features

- May be asymptomatic or cause paraesthesia in the nerve distribution.
- May be multiple in people with hereditary neurofibromatosis (Figure 2.4).
- Occasionally undergo malignant change when they become an aggressive type of sarcoma called a malignant peripheral nerve sheath tumour (MPNST). This is very rare and may be indicated by rapid enlargement or pain.

> **MICRO-print**
> Von Recklinghausen's disease (also known as neurofibromatosis type I) is an inherited condition where there are multiple congenital neurofibromata.

2.3.6 HAEMANGIOMA

- These are benign tumours composed of abnormal blood vessels.
- There are a number of different types. Some occur in infancy, others in later life.
  - They are the most common tumour in infancy.
    - Usually appear during the first weeks of life.
    - May resolve by age 10.

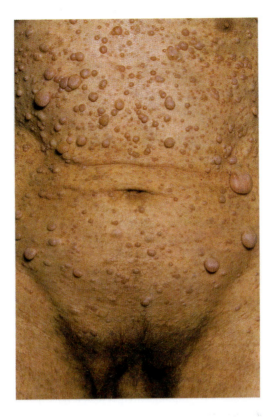

Figure 2.4 Multiple neurofibromatosis. (From: *Browse's Introduction to the Symptoms and Signs of Surgical Disease, 4th Edition*, Figure 3.)

Clinical features

- 80% are located on the face and neck.
- Their appearance may vary.
  - When on the surface of the skin they resemble a ripe strawberry (hence strawberry haemangioma).
  - When just under the skin they are merely a bluish swelling.

Treatment

- Usually treated conservatively unless disfiguring.
- Topical corticosteroids have been used.
- Laser therapy may be successful if small.
- Surgical excision.
- Embolisation may be suitable for some lesions with obvious feeding vessels.

2.3.7 LYMPHADENOPATHY

- Lymph nodes, with the spleen, tonsils, thymus gland and Peyer's patches, are organised centres of immune cells that filter antigen from the extracellular fluid.
- Enlarged lymph nodes (lymphadenopathy) are a common diagnostic problem, for which there is a long differential diagnosis.
- When assessing lymphadenopathy there are several considerations:
  - Is it localised (isolated to one regional nodal group) or generalised (involving more than one regional nodal group)?
  - The character of the glands:
    - Size.
      - >1 cm is generally considered abnormal.
    - Location.
      - What are the draining regions?
    - Consistency.
      - Stony hard may suggest malignancy.
      - Firm and rubbery may suggest lymphoma.
      - Soft may indicate infection or inflammation.
      - Fluctuant nodes are likely to be suppurated.
      - Matted nodes are often indicative of TB or malignancy.
    - Tenderness.
      - Indicates a rapid increase in size with stretch of the capsule.
  - Associated signs or symptoms, particularly:
    - Obvious source of infection, inflammation or malignancy?
    - Constitutional symptoms (weight loss, fever, night sweats, malaise and myalgia)?
    - Presence of hepatosplenomegaly?
    - Epidemiological clues (e.g. foreign travel or high-risk behaviour)?
    - Age of the patient (malignancy is far commoner >50 years of age)?
- Core or excision biopsy is recommended, rather than fine-needle aspiration (FNA), as the lymph node architecture is preserved, allowing diagnosis of lymphoma if appropriate.
- A diagnostic algorithm for lymphadenopathy is shown in Figure 2.5.

MICRO-facts

Lymph node drainage:
- Cervical: Oropharynx, head, trachea.
- Right supraclavicular: Mediastinum, lungs, upper 2/3 oesophagus.
- Left supraclavicular: Thorax, abdomen via thoracic duct.
- Axilla: Arm, chest wall, breast.
- Inguinal: Lower limbs, genitalia (excluding testes), perineum, anal canal, lower abdominal wall.
- Para-aortic: Testes, abdomen.

General surgery

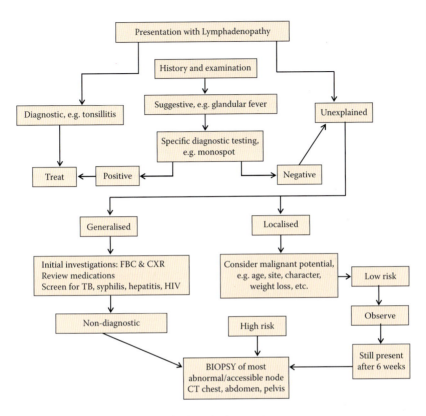

Figure 2.5 Diagnostic algorithm for lymphadenopathy.

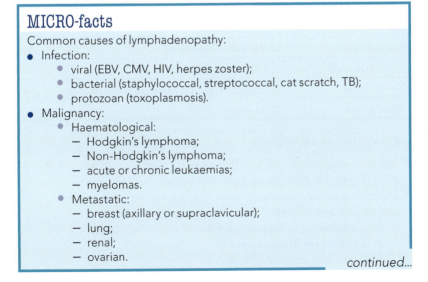

MICRO-facts

Common causes of lymphadenopathy:
- Infection:
  - viral (EBV, CMV, HIV, herpes zoster);
  - bacterial (staphylococcal, streptococcal, cat scratch, TB);
  - protozoan (toxoplasmosis).
- Malignancy:
  - Haematological:
    - Hodgkin's lymphoma;
    - Non-Hodgkin's lymphoma;
    - acute or chronic leukaemias;
    - myelomas.
  - Metastatic:
    - breast (axillary or supraclavicular);
    - lung;
    - renal;
    - ovarian.

continued...

continued...

- Hypersensitivity:
  - Drugs (allopurinol, atenolol, captopril, carbamazepine, cephalosporins, penicillin, phenytoin, sulphonamides).
  - Silicone (e.g. in breast implants).
- Connective tissue disease:
  - rheumatoid arthritis;
  - systemic lupus erythematosis.
- Other:
  - Sarcoidosis.

2.4 MALIGNANT SOFT TISSUE SWELLINGS

2.4.1 DEFINITION

- A sarcoma is a cancer arising from tissues that were derived from the embryonic mesoderm (muscle, fat, bone, cartilage) rather than the ectoderm (skin, viscera, epithelia of all types).
- Cancers arising from epithelia are called carcinomas and are vastly more common than sarcomas.
  - Sarcomas account for only 1% of all malignancies in the UK.
- Named after type of tissue from which they arise, there are over 150 different types of sarcoma (see Table 2.1).

Table 2.1 Sarcoma names based on tissue of origin.

TISSUE OF ORIGIN	TUMOUR NAME
Bone	Osteosarcoma
Cartilage	Chondrosarcoma
Fat	Liposarcoma
Striated muscle	Rhabdomyosarcoma
Smooth muscle	Leiomyosarcoma
Nerve sheath	Malignant peripheral nerve sheath tumour
Blood vessel	Angiosarcoma

2.4.2 CLINICAL FEATURES

- The presenting symptom is usually a mass that may arise anywhere in the body (Figure 2.6 shows an example on the thigh).
- Depending on the anatomic location, the tumour may cause pain or neurological symptoms by:
  - Compressing or stretching nerves.
  - Irritating overlying bursae.
  - Expanding sensitive structures.

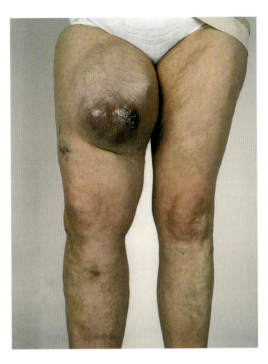

Figure 2.6 A large rhabdomyosarcoma arising from the quadriceps muscle. (*Browse's Introduction to the Symptoms and Signs of Surgical Disease, 4th Edition*, Figure 4.6.)

MICRO-facts

Features that favour a malignant, rather than benign, lesion:
- Rapid increase in size.
- Masses larger than 5 cm in diameter.
- Lesions arising from deeper, rather than subcutaneous tissues.
- Adherence to adjacent structures.
- Pain.

2.4.3 STAGING

- Graded as high, low or intermediate, based on size, anatomic location and histological grade of differentiation (see Table 2.2).

2.4.4 TREATMENT

- The treatment of sarcomas is highly specialised and all suspected cases should be referred to 1 of the 3 national bone sarcoma units or 1 of the 15 national soft tissue sarcoma units for further management.

General surgery

Table 2.2 UICC staging system for soft tissue sarcomas.

STAGE	GRADE	TUMOUR	NODES	METASTASES
IA	Low grade	T1a–T1b Small: Superficial or deep	N0	M0
IB	Low grade	T2a Large: Superficial	N0	M0
IIA	Low grade	T2b Large: Deep	N0	M0
IIB	High grade	T1a–T1b Small: Superficial or deep	N0	M0
IIC	High grade	T2a Large: Superficial	N0	M0
III	High grade	T2b Large: Deep	N0	M0
IV	Any G	Any T	N0/N1	M0/M1

N.B. Large is defined as >5 cm, small as <5 cm.

- For most common variants, such as liposarcomas, leoimyosarcomas, myxofibrosarcomas or undifferentiated sarcomas, treatment is preceded by detailed imaging of the lesion with magnetic resonance imaging (MRI) to assess operability and CT scanning to confirm the absence of lung metastases (the most common metastatic site).
    - Treatment is then surgical excision, ideally with a margin of normal surrounding tissue.
    - For larger or higher-grade lesions, post-operative radiotherapy is given.
    - Most sarcomas are very resistant to chemotherapy, and so there is no role for post-operative or adjuvant chemotherapy.
- There are some special types of sarcomas that are highly chemosensitive, such that chemotherapy is the first-line treatment, with surgery just used to remove any residual disease after chemotherapy has finished.
    - These include Ewing's sarcoma, rhabdomyosarcoma and osteosarcoma, all of which are most common in teenagers and young adults.

MICRO-print
Limb conservation is now the rule rather than the exception in sarcoma surgery. Thirty years ago all limb sarcomas were treated with amputation, but careful research has shown that good quality surgery to achieve a margin around the tumour, with the use of post-operative radiotherapy when indicated, achieves equivalent survival rates.

2.4.5 PROGNOSIS

- Higher-grade tumours are more likely to undergo metastasis (which is most commonly to the lungs). Unlike in some tumours where metastatic disease is incurable, selected cases of sarcoma, with limited, operable lung metastases, may achieve good long-term survival following lung metastasectomy.
- Increasing size of primary tumour is associated with a poorer prognosis.
  - Wide local excision (WLE) of small, superficial, low-grade tumours has a very low risk of recurrence.
- Site is another important prognostic factor, with superficial tumours (above and separate from the muscular fascia) having a better prognosis than those that involve deep fascias.

2.5 HOW TO EXAMINE A SOFT TISSUE SWELLING

2.5.1 EXAMINATION SEQUENCE

- Introduce yourself and ask permission to examine.
- Ensure a chaperone is present.
- Clean your hands.
- Ask if the area to be examined is painful.
- Adequately expose the area.
- Inspect for differences in colour or texture of the overlying skin.

MICRO-facts

Features to note in a lump:
- Size.
- Position.
- Attachments.
- Surface.
- Edge.
- Consistency.
- Transillumination.
- Colour.
- Temperature.
- Thrills, bruits, noises.

- Palpation.
  - Is there tenderness?
  - Assess temperature.
  - Define the site and shape.
  - Examine the edge of the swelling.
    - A well-demarcated edge is more likely to be benign.
    - An indefinite margin may suggest infiltrating malignancy.

- Can you feel all the edges?
- Measure its size (enables more accurate assessment of any change).
- Examine for a pulse.
  - Aneurysms will be expansile.
  - Highly vascular tumours may transmit a palpable pulse.
- Attempt to pick up the overlying skin—is it attached?
- Try and move the lump in different planes—is it attached to deep tissues?
- Assess consistency.
  - Hard swellings are more likely to suggest malignancy or calcification.
  - Soft swellings are less likely to be malignant.
- Elicit any fluctuance (presence of fluid) by compressing the swelling on one side and visualising/feeling a bulge on the other side.
- Auscultate for any bruits or bowel sounds.
- Transilluminate (cystic lesions will transmit light).

2.6 SUPERFICIAL INFECTIONS

2.6.1 BOIL

- Also known as a furuncle.
- Definition: Infected hair follicle.
- Usual organism: *Staphylococcus aureus*.

Associations

- Immunosuppression.
- Diabetes mellitus.

> **MICRO-facts**
>
> In patients presenting with recurrent infections, check the blood sugar to rule out undiagnosed diabetes.

Prognosis

- Usually self-limiting but may progress to form an abscess with surrounding cellulitis and generalised septicaemia.

Treatment

- Usually none but may require treatment if progresses to abscess formation.

> **MICRO-print**
>
> Pus has two phases: solid (polymorphs, macrophages, bacteria, cells from involved tissues, fibrin meshwork) and liquid (immunoglobulins, complement, clotting cascade factors, kinins, cytokines).

2.6.2 ABSCESS

- An abscess is a localised collection of pus.

Clinical features

- Red, painful lump.
- Pus may 'point' at the skin.
- There may be generalised sepsis.

Treatment

- Antibiotics.
- Incision and drainage (I&D) with the wound left open to heal by secondary intention so pus doesn't recollect.
- Improve diabetic control.

2.6.3 HIDRANITITIS SUPPRATIVA

- This is infection of the apocrine sweat glands.
- The usual causative organism is *Staphylococcus aureus*; rarely *Coliforms* may be responsible.

Clinical features (see Figure 2.7)

- Occurs in the axillae, groin, perineum, perianal and infra-mammary areas.
- Affected area is indurated and inflamed with sinuses containing pus.
- Often initially misdiagnosed as recurrent abscesses, boils, or perianal fistulae.

Treatment

- Weight loss.
- Loose-fitting clothes.

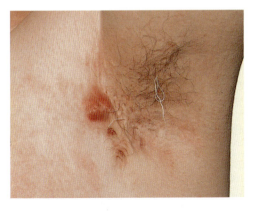

Figure 2.7 Hidradenitis supprativa. (From: *Browse's Introduction to the Symptoms and Signs of Surgical Disease, 4th Edition*, Figure 3.22.)

General surgery

- Improve regional hygiene.
- Antibiotics for acute infections.
  - Low-dose prophylactic antibiotics may also be required in recurrent cases.
- I&D if abscess forms (send roof for histology to confirm diagnosis).
- Severe cases may require WLE ± skin grafting.
- In severe perianal disease treatment may include diverting colostomy before skin grafting.

2.7 SKIN CANCERS

2.7.1 BASAL CELL CARCINOMA (BCC)

- Definition: A malignant lesion of the basal cells of the epidermis.
- Also known as a rodent ulcer.

Epidemiology

- Commonest malignant skin tumour.
- More common in elderly men (M:F = 2:1).
- Higher incidence in areas of high UV exposure, e.g. Australia.

Aetiology

- High association with exposure to UV light.
- Association with exposure to irradiation.

> **MICRO-facts**
>
> **Distinguishing point:** BCC is rare on the ear, whereas SCC is common on the ear.

Clinical features (see Figure 2.8)

- Common sites:
  - peri-orbital;
  - naso-labial folds;
  - scalp hairline;
  - rare on ear.
  - 90% occur superior to the line joining the angle of the mouth to the external auditory meatus.
- Appearance:
  - pearl-coloured;
  - raised, rolled edges;
  - central depression;
  - telangiectasia over lesion;
- Presents as a slow-growing papule/nodule.

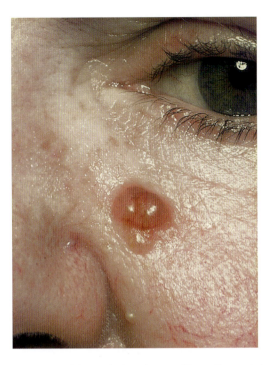

Figure 2.8 An early BCC nodule just below the eye. (From: *Browse's Introduction to the Symptoms and Signs of Surgical Disease, 4th Edition*, Figure 3.41.)

- Usually early presentation due to high visibility of site.
- Often multiple.
- Can ulcerate (hence the term *rodent ulcer*).

Diagnosis
- Usually on clinical grounds and may be confirmed by excision biopsy.

Treatment
- Depends on:
  - location;.
  - size;
  - clinical and histological appearance;
  - patient choice.
- Cryotherapy if small.
- Usually local surgical excision with a 3–5 mm margin.
- Radiotherapy.
- Photodynamic therapy.
- Topical chemotherapy (5-fluorouracil or imiquimod).

- Curettage and electrocautery, especially if older.
- Mohs micrographic surgery if recurrent.

Prognosis
- Usually excellent.
- Rarely fatal.
- Almost never metastasises but may erode into local structures.

> **MICRO-reference**
> *The management of low-risk basal cell carcinomas in the community* (2010). London: National Institute for Health and Clinical Excellence.

2.7.2 SQUAMOUS CELL CARCINOMA (SCC)
- Definition: A malignant lesion of the keratinocytes of the epidermis.
- Also known as epithelioma.

Epidemiology
- Second commonest malignant skin tumour.
- More common in elderly men (M:F = 2:1).
- Higher incidence in Caucasians living in the tropics.

Aetiology
- Exposure to:
    - UV light;
    - ionizing radiation;
    - industrial carcinogens, e.g. tar, soot, arsenic, mineral oils.
- Infection with human papilloma virus (HPV) strains 6, 11, 16 or 18.
- Immunosuppression.
- Chronic irritation.
- Chronic ulceration.

Clinical features (see Figure 2.9)
- Common sites:
    - exposed areas of face, including the ear;
    - backs of hands;
    - HPV-associated sites (mouth and tongue, anal glands, glans penis, cervix).
- Appearance:
    - usually exophytic growth;
    - indurating, rolled margins;

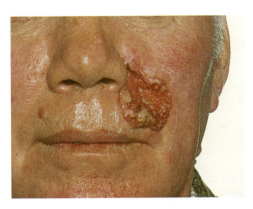

Figure 2.9 An SCC on the face—note the ulcer has an everted edge and necrotic base. (From: *Browse's Introduction to the Symptoms and Signs of Surgical Disease, 4th Edition*, Figure 3.42.)

- central necrosis;
- ulceration;
- bleeding.
- Painless, rapid growth.

> **MICRO-print**
> A *Marjolin's ulcer* is an ulcerating SCC in an area of chronic irritation, particularly after a burn.

Diagnosis

- Excision biopsy.
- FNA or biopsy of lymph nodes if involvement suspected.
- CT/MRI imaging if distant metastases suspected.

Treatment

- Surgical excision is the mainstay of treatment.
- Radiotherapy.
- Chemotherapy (5-fluorouracil) if multiple early lesions.
- Block dissection of lymph nodes is indicated if lymph node involvement.

Prognosis

- May be locally destructive.
- Will spread to regional lymph nodes in 5–10%.
- Distant metastases are uncommon.
- Overall prognosis following treatment is usually excellent.
- Follow-up for 5 years following treatment.

General surgery

2.7.3 MALIGNANT MELANOMA (MM)

Definition: A malignant lesion of the melanocytes.

Epidemiology

- Third commonest tumour in the 15–39 year age group.
- Peak incidence in the fourth decade.
- M = F.
- Accounts for 10% of all skin cancers.
- 80% are seen in Caucasian individuals.

> **MICRO-reference**
> *Improving outcomes for people with skin tumours including melanoma: The manual* (2006). London: National Institute for Health and Clinical Excellence.

Aetiology

- High UV exposure.
- High susceptibility to sunburn (i.e. blonde/red hair, blue eyes, fair skin, freckling or albinism).
- Sunburn at a young age or severe sunburn, i.e. blistering.
- Solar keratosis.
- Dysplastic naevus syndrome.
- Congenital hairy naevi.
- Personal or family history of MM.

Clinical features (see Figure 2.10)

- Can occur anywhere but common sites include:
  - back in males;
  - legs in females.

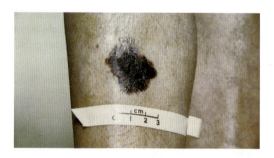

Figure 2.10 A superficial spreading malignant melanoma. Note the thin lesion with an irregular edge and varying pigmentation. (From: *Browse's Introduction to the Symptoms and Signs of Surgical Disease*, 4th Edition, Figure 3.44.)

> ## MICRO-facts
> 5 changes to watch for in a mole:
> **A**—Asymmetry.
> **B**—Border irregularity.
> **C**—Colour variegation.
> **D**—Diameter > 6 mm.
> **E**—Elevation.

- Usually presents as a change in a pigmented lesion:
  - increase in size;
  - change in pigmentation strength or consistency;
  - spreading of pigmentation (irregular borders);
  - bleeding;
  - ulceration;
  - pain.
- Satellite lesions.
- Lymphadenopathy.
- There are four common subtypes of melanoma (see Table 2.3).

> ## MICRO-facts
> Remember the subtypes using the mnemonic:
> **Several** = **S**uperficial spreading.
> **New** = **N**odular melanoma.
> **Lesions or moles** = **L**entigo**m**aligna melanoma.
> **Appearing** = **A**cral melanoma.

Staging
- Uses the tumour, nodes, metastases (TNM) classification.
- Relies on the Breslow depth of tumour thickness.
- Use of Clark's levels to describe the location of the tumour within skin layers is less accurate, so less commonly done.

Metastatic spread
- Unpredictable.
- Via lymphatics initially, then later haematological spread.
- Common sites:
  - lungs;
  - liver;
  - brain;
  - bone.
- Free melanin within the bloodstream can lead to generalised pigmentation.

Table 2.3 Subtypes of malignant melanoma.

Superficial spreading	70% of melanoma. Spreading of existing naevus. Large and flat. Deep irregular pigmentation. Lateral growth precedes vertical invasion.
Nodular melanoma	10% of melanoma. Rapidly growing pigmented nodule. May bleed or ulcerate. Vertical growth. Can be amelanotic (5%). Most aggressive type. Earlier lymphatic involvement. Commoner in men.
Lentigomaligna melanoma	7% of melanoma. Malignant change of lentigomaligna (pale facial lesion). Darkly pigmented papule or nodule. Usually seen on cheeks. Good prognosis. Commoner in elderly women.
Acrallentiginous melanoma	13% of melanoma. Pigmented lesions on palms, soles or under nails. Usually presents late; therefore poor prognosis. Commoner in black individuals.

Diagnosis

- Excision biopsy.
- Refer any suspicious lesions urgently under the 2-week-wait rule.
- CT for metastases if stage II lesion or higher.

Treatment

- Surgery is the mainstay of treatment.
- Adjuvant therapies:
  - no survival benefit with chemotherapy;
  - no clear survival benefit with radiotherapy or immunotherapy.
- Localised disease:
  - Wide excision with margins according to depth of tumour.
    - Cover of excision site with either primary closure or the use of rotational flaps—refer to plastic surgery.

- Sentinel lymph node biopsy (SLNB) if tumour ≥ 1mm.
- Radical lymph node dissection if SLNB is positive.

MICRO-print

Surgical margins according to Breslow thickness:

- In situ tumour = 5 mm.
- <1 mm tumour = 1 cm.
- 1.1–2 mm tumour = 1–2 cm.
- 2.1–4 mm tumour = 2–3 cm.
- >4 mm tumour = 3 cm.

- Loco-regional recurrent disease:
  - Wide local excision.
  - If progressive consider chemotherapy.
  - If poorly controlled consider radiotherapy.
- Metastatic disease:
  - MDT approach;
  - palliation using surgery, chemotherapy and radiotherapy as appropriate.

MICRO-reference

Marsden JR et al. Revised UK guidelines for the management of cutaneous melanoma 2010. *British Journal of Dermatology* 2010; 163: 238–256.

Prognosis

- 5-year survival = 73% (males), 85% (females).
- Biggest prognostic indicator is Breslow thickness.
- Poor prognostic factors:
  - increasing thickness of tumour;
  - increasing stage of tumour;
  - acral or nodular subtype;
  - presence of satellite lesions;
  - head or truncal lesions;
  - ulceration of primary lesion.

Prevention

- Avoid excess sun exposure, especially at the hottest part of the day.
- Avoid using sun beds.

General surgery

MICRO-facts

Poorer prognostic signs for SCC:
- Located on ear, lip or non-sun-exposed sites, e.g. perineum.
- In pre-existing scars.
- Immunosuppression.
- Greater than 4 mm depth.
- Greater than 2 cm in diameter.
- Poor differentiation of tumour.
- Perineural invasion.

3 Breast

- The relations of the female breast are shown in Figure 3.1.

3.1 BREAST EXAMINATION

- Examination of the female breast is a sensitive and highly personal experience; respect, privacy and sensitivity should be maintained at all times.
- A female chaperone should **always** be present, and there should be a gown available to cover the patient once the examination is complete.

3.1.1 EXAMINATION SEQUENCE

- Introduce yourself.
- Clean your hands.
- Ask whether the breasts are tender and identify any particular tender areas if present.
- Explain what you are going to do at each stage of the procedure.

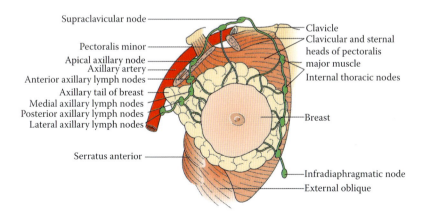

Figure 3.1 The female breast with its relations and lymphatic drainage. (From: *Illustrated Clinical Anatomy, 2nd Edition*, Figure 1.15, p. 30.)

Inspection

- Inspect the breasts from the front with the patient in each of the three positions shown in Figure 3.2.
  - Resting the hands at the patient's sides with her sitting upright relaxes the pectoral muscles, allowing assessment of symmetry.
  - Placing the hands above and behind the head stretches the pectoral muscles and skin over the breast.
  - Pushing in with hands on the hips contracts the pectoral muscles, revealing any tethering or distortion.
- Look for asymmetry, swelling, change in skin contour or nipple retraction.

Diseases of the breast and their assessment and treatment

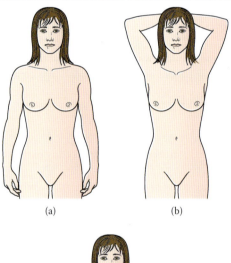

(a)   (b)

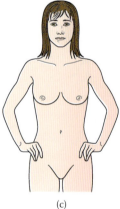

(c)

Figure 3.2 Positions for inspection of the breasts. (From: *Obstetrics, Gynaecology, and Women's Health on the Move*, Figure 20.2 (a-c), p. 256.)

Palpation

- The patient should be lying on a couch at 45° with her head supported with a pillow and her hands placed behind her head if she has large pendulous breasts or by her sides if she has smaller breasts.
- Using the flat of your fingers, systematically examine all quadrants of the breast, including the area behind the nipple and the axillary tail.
- Elicit any areas of tenderness or thickening and identify any discrete lumps, noting the size, position, mobility, consistency and whether it is fixed to the chest wall or skin.
- If you are unable to find the lump, ask the patient to find it for you and examine again.

Lymph node examination (see Figure 3.3)

- To examine the axillae the patient's corresponding arm should be fully supported using your non-examining arm in order to relax the muscles.
- Using the flat of your hand, compress the axillary contents against the chest wall, feeling for any palpable masses.
- The supraclavicular fossae should also be palpated to detect any palpable nodes.
- Thank the patient and ask her to sit up.
- If cancer is suspected, you may also wish to examine for hepatomegaly, pleural effusion and spinal tenderness.
- Remember to cover the patient with an appropriate gown when you have finished the examination.

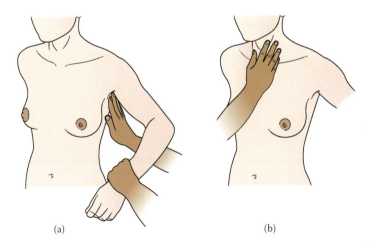

(a) (b)

Figure 3.3 Examination of axillary and supraclavicular lymph nodes. (From: *Obstetrics, Gynaecology, and Women's Health on the Move*, Figure 20.3, p. 258.)

General surgery

3.2 BENIGN BREAST DISEASES

- All presentations of breast disease should be seen in a fast-track clinic with the facility to perform triple assessment.
- The majority of all referrals to the breast clinic are with benign disease, such as hormonal nodularity, cysts, cyclical mastalgia and nipple discharge.
  - Only 1 in 10 new breast clinic appointments are with women who have cancer (but this number increases in older women).
- Common presentations to the breast clinic include a palpable lump or asymmetrical thickening, pain, nipple discharge and change in breast shape. Each should be assessed individually, in the context of age, hormone status and family history.
- In women under the age of 35, the imaging of choice is ultrasound scan (USS); women over 35 will undergo mammography plus USS of any lumps.

3.2.1 BENIGN BREAST CHANGE

- Often referred to as fibrocystic change or benign breast change.
- It is cyclical nodularity and pain in pre-menopausal women.

Clinical features

- Pain and nodularity changes that may undergo cyclical variation.

Management

- Reassurance that symptoms will often resolve spontaneously.
- Simple analgesia (e.g. paracetamol) if required.
- Any area of asymmetric nodularity must be subjected to triple assessment.

> ## MICRO-facts
>
> Indications for imaging assessment include:
> - New discrete lump.
> - Asymmetrical nodularity or thickening.
> - Focal breast pain.
> - Palpable axillary lump.
> - Breast cellulitis.
> - Nipple discharge.

3.2.2 FIBROADENOMA

- Sometimes referred to as a breast mouse due to the small size and mobility.
- They are benign breast tumours of hyperplastic fibrous and glandular tissue.
- Fibroadenomas account for 13% of all breast lumps.
- They are commonest in women of child-bearing age (aged 20–40 years).

Clinical features

- Painless, firm, mobile breast lump with a clearly defined border.
- They are oestrogen responsive, so may be associated with cyclical pain.
- Increase in size during pregnancy.

Diagnosis

- Triple assessment, including core biopsy, as phylloides tumours can occasionally be mistaken for fibroadenoma on USS alone.

Management

- Excision is only recommended if >3 cm in diameter or if the histological diagnosis is not certain.

MICRO-case

A 24-year-old woman presents with a 1 cm firm, discrete lump in her right breast. She noticed it whilst washing. It has not changed in size. On examination you can feel a smooth, mobile lump. There are no overlying skin changes and the rest of the examination is normal. USS confirms the typical appearance of a fibroadenoma and a core biopsy confirms this.

Learning points:

- Despite its classical presentation, fibroadenomata should always be confirmed histologically, as they have a similar appearance to phylloides tumours, even in young women.
- Treatment is reassurance.
  - 10% increase in size and should be reassessed.
  - 30% decrease in size and may disappear.
  - 60% remain the same.

3.2.3 BREAST CYSTS

- Breast cysts are distended fluid-filled breast lobules.
- They are commonest in peri-menopausal women (aged 40–55 years).

Clinical features

- Smooth, discrete breast lump.
- May be associated with pain or tenderness.

Diagnosis

- Triple assessment with a halo on mammography and fluid-filled on USS.

Management

- Aspiration under USS guidance—fluid may be clear, green or brownish.

- May be associated with a cancer; features requiring further investigation include:
  - blood-stained aspirate;
  - persistence of lump following aspiration or repeated refilling;
  - irregular or thickened wall on imaging.

3.2.4 FAT NECROSIS

Aetiology
- Results from trauma, although only 40% recall the preceding trauma.

Clinical features
- A firm, mobile mass with a clearly defined border.
- Breast pain or bruising.

Diagnosis
- Triple assessment with USS or mammography and biopsy.

Management
- Reassurance that symptoms will resolve with conservative treatment.
- Simple analgesia if required.

3.2.5 BREAST ABSCESS

Aetiology
- In breast-feeding women this is due to blockage of the ducts with subsequent inflammation (mastitis) and bacterial infection.
  - Usual causative bacterium is *Staphylococcus aureus*.
- Non-lactational abscess are usually due to periductal mastitis or duct ectasia.
  - Usual causative bacterium is *Streptococcus* spp.
  - Common in smokers.

Clinical features
- Painful swelling in the breast, often associated with overlying cellulitis.
- May have associated systemic features of infection.

Diagnosis
- Confirmed by USS or aspiration.

Management
- Antibiotic therapy.
  - Flucloxacillin in lactating women (erythromycin if penicillin allergic).
  - Co-amoxiclav in non-lactating women.

- Aspiration of pus is preferable to formal incision and drainage initially.
- Surgical incision and drainage may be required in unresponsive or progressive cases, if there is multi-loculation or overlying skin necrosis.

> **MICRO-case**
> A 34-year-old breast-feeding woman presents with a painful, red breast lump. She has features of systemic infection, with fever and malaise. USS confirms a breast abscess and she is commenced on flucloxacillin and undergoes aspiration of the abscess under USS guidance.
> **Learning points:**
> - Aspiration of pus in combination with antibiotics will result in resolution in most cases; incision and drainage is rarely required.
> - Pus should be sent for culture to guide antibiotic therapy.
> - Lactational abscesses usually occur in the first 6 weeks of breast feeding and are due to cracked nipples acting as a portal for bacteria.

3.2.6 GYNAECOMASTIA

- Enlargement of the male breast due to hyperplasia of the ductal epithelium and proliferation of peri-ductal stroma or excess fat deposition.
- May be unilateral or bilateral.

Aetiology

- Physiological (neonatal, pubertal and elderly).
- Drugs (cannabis, anabolic steroids, spironolactone, anti-androgens).
- Alcohol excess.
- Liver failure.
- Klinefelter syndrome.
- Tumours (testicular, pituitary, adrenal).
- Obesity.

Diagnosis

- Confirmed with USS but may require core biopsy and or mammography.

Management

- Treat the underlying cause.
- Reassurance that there is no breast cancer and that enlargement will often regress in time.
- Subcutaneous mastectomy.
  - Should be performed by a specialist breast or plastic surgeon.

General surgery

3.3 BREAST CANCER

3.3.1 EPIDEMIOLOGY

- Breast cancer is the most common cancer diagnosed in women in the UK, affecting over 40,000 women and resulting in 13,000 deaths per year.
- 1 in 8 women will develop breast cancer in their lifetime.
- Peak incidence is in the seventh decade.

3.3.2 AETIOLOGY

- Aetiological factors for the development of breast cancer are shown in Figure 3.4).

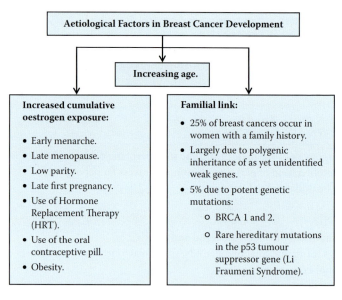

Figure 3.4 Aetiological factors associated with breast cancer development.

3.3.3 CLINICAL FEATURES

- Painless lump in the breast.
- Distortion or tethering of the breast tissue or overlying skin (as seen in Figure 3.5).
- Peau d'orange (skin oedema caused by dermal lymphatic infiltration).
- Nipple retraction or inversion (as seen in Figure 3.5).
- Nipple discharge, especially if blood-stained.
- Asymmetric breast nodularity.
- Paget's disease of the nipple (looks very much like eczema).
- May also present with signs of metastatic disease in 5% of cases:

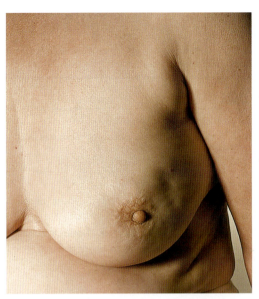

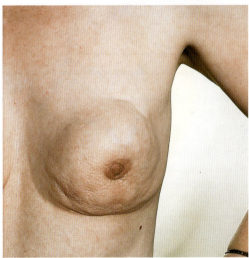

Figure 3.5 Patient with breast cancer demonstrating nipple retraction and puckering/tethering of the skin. (From: *Browse's Introduction to Symptoms & Signs of Surgical Disease, 4th Edition*, Figure 12.4, p. 320.)

- pathological fractures;
- bone pain;
- jaundice;
- cough or breathlessness.
- May be asymptomatic at presentation.

> ## MICRO-facts
> 30% of all UK breast cancers are diagnosed by the NHS Breast Screening Programme in women with no symptoms or signs.

3.3.4 DIAGNOSIS

- Diagnosis is by triple assessment (Figure 3.6).
- Other tests may be indicated once triple assessment has been performed. These may include:
  - Breast MRI to look for multi-focality, lobular cancer, or assess disease extent in women with breast implants.
  - In women with signs of more advanced cancer (nodal disease or locally advanced):
    - CT scan to stage for lung, liver and bone metastases;
    - isotope bone scan to stage for bone metastases.

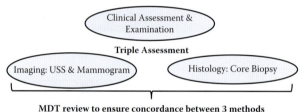

Figure 3.6 Components of triple assessment.

3.3.5 HISTOLOGICAL GRADING

- Graded from 1 to 3 based on degree of:
  - gland acinus formation;
  - nuclear pleomorphism;
  - mitosis count.
- Higher grades are associated with increased risk of distant metastatic spread, decreased cancer-specific survival and decreased disease-free survival.

3.3.6 TUMOUR RECEPTOR STATUS

- Breast cancer cells may express two different cellular receptors that have both prognostic and therapeutic significance: ER and HER2 (Figure 3.7).

ER (Oestrogen Receptor)	HER 2 (Epidermal Growth Factor Receptor, Type 2)
70% of breast cancers express this.	30% of breast cancers express this.

Figure 3.7 Cellular receptors expressed by breast cancers.

> **MICRO-print**
> Some cancers express both receptors and some neither. The latter are
> called triple negative cancers (they also do not express the
> progesterone receptor). Triple negative cancers are sometimes linked to
> the BRCA 1 gene mutation and have a poor prognosis.

3.3.7 STAGING

- Breast cancer staging is by the tumour, nodes, metastases (TNM) staging
  system (Table 3.1).

Table 3.1 TNM staging for breast cancer.

PRIMARY TUMOUR (T)		LYMPH NODE STATUS (N)		METASTASES (M)	
Tx	Primary tumour cannot be assessed.	Nx	Unable to assess lymph node status.	Mx	Unable to assess for metastases.
T0	No evidence of primary tumour.	N0	No evidence of lymph node spread.	M0	No evidence of metastasis.
Tis	Carcinoma in situ. DCIS: ductal. LCIS: lobular. Paget's disease with no invasive component.	N1	Metastasis in moveable axillary lymph nodes.	M1	Metastatic spread.
T1	Tumour ≤ 2 cm in greatest dimension.	N2	Metastasis in fixed axillary lymph nodes ± internal mammary nodes.		
T2	Tumour ≥ 2 cm, <5 cm.	N3	Metastasis in supraclavicular lymph nodes ± axillary/ internal mammary nodes.		
T3	Tumour > 5 cm.				
T4	Tumour of any size with direct invasion into chest wall or skin.				

> **MICRO-facts**
>
> Several factors must be taken in to account in breast cancer management:
> - Stage of the tumour.
> - Size of the tumour in relation to the breast.
> - Receptor status (including ER and HER-2).
> - The wishes of the patient.
> - The fitness of the patient.

3.3.8 MANAGEMENT

Surgery

- The primary treatment modality for breast cancer in most women with operable disease is surgery. This takes two main forms: breast conservation surgery and mastectomy.
- Breast conservation surgery (wide local excision).
  - The tumour is excised with a 0.5–1 cm margin of normal breast tissue.
  - Up to 20% of breast volume may be removed without causing significant distortion.
  - Breast reshaping may be required to reduce distortion.
  - Post-operative radiotherapy is given to the affected breast.
  - 10–12% 20-year recurrence rates.

> **MICRO-facts**
>
> Indications for mastectomy:
> - Large tumour relative to breast size.
> - Multi-focal tumour.
> - Previous breast radiotherapy.
> - Patient choice.

- Mastectomy.
  - Excision of the entire breast.
  - Standard mastectomy may be used, which includes removal of a skin ellipse across the whole width of the breast.
  - Skin-sparing mastectomy may be performed (through a range of incisions to retain more skin and even the nipple), with immediate reconstruction. This gives enhanced cosmetic outcomes.
  - All women who undergo mastectomy should be considered for breast reconstruction, although only 15% of women will choose to have a reconstruction.
  - The majority of women who have a mastectomy have a breast prosthesis to wear inside their bra to restore clothed cosmesis.

- For those who want reconstruction there may be several options:
  - Delayed or immediate, depending on the need for further treatment and patient wishes.
  - Silicone implant-based reconstruction may be used, either immediately or following tissue expansion.
  - Autogenous reconstruction involves transfer of a flap of skin, muscle and fat from a donor site, such as the back or abdomen.

MICRO-print

Types of flaps:

- Pedicle flap (e.g. latissimus dorsi).
- Free flap (e.g. transverse rectus abdominis myocutaneous (TRAM) flap) using microsurgery to re-anastomose divided blood vessels.

- Axillary lymph node surgery.
  - Axillary node biopsy is required in all patients with invasive breast cancer.
  - Pre-operative imaging and biopsy of abnormal nodes is performed on all patients and identifies >50% of those who have nodal spread.
  - Axillary node sampling removes four nodes from the affected axilla.
    - The false negative rate is ~5%.
    - Arm lymphoedema rate of 1–2%.
  - Sentinel lymph node biopsy involves injection of blue dye (Figure 3.8) and radioactive tracer into the breast tissue. This drains into the lymphatic supply, allowing identification of lymph nodes due to either their blue colour or via an intra-operative Gieger counter.

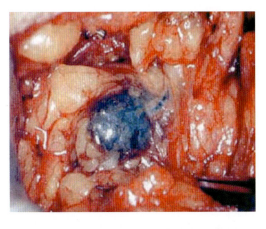

Figure 3.8 Blue lymphatic channel and lymph node. (From: *Browse's Introduction to the Investigation and Management of Surgical Disease*, Figure 5.12, p. 96.)

General surgery

- The false negative rate is also ~5%.
- Arm lymphoedema rate of 1–2%.
- Axillary node clearance is performed if there is confirmed metastatic lymph node spread.
  - It may be done at the time of primary surgery if pre-operative staging with US and biopsy confirms nodal disease, or a second procedure may be needed at a later date if axillary sampling/sentinel node biopsy confirms nodal spread.
  - It involves removal of all axillary tissue up to the level of the axillary vein.
  - It is associated with a 15% risk of arm lymphoedema, which is why it is not performed routinely on all women with breast cancer.

Adjuvant therapies

- Many women are offered additional therapies to help reduce the risk of recurrence (see Table 3.2).
- Decisions regarding adjuvant therapies are made in conjunction with the MDT, based on the stage and biology of the disease and the patient's tolerances and wishes.
- Radiotherapy.

Table 3.2 Comparison of adjuvant therapies.

RADIOTHERAPY	CHEMOTHERAPY	ANTI-OESTROGEN THERAPY	ANTI-HER2 THERAPY
All patients having breast conservation surgery.	Patients with aggressive tumours.	All patients with ER positive tumours.	All patients with HER2 positive tumours.
↓ recurrence rates from ~35% to 10–12%.	↓ recurrence and mortality (depending on tumour characteristics).	↓ recurrence rates by ~25% and death by 17%.	↓ mortality rates by 34% compared to chemotherapy alone.
Every day for 3–5 days.	6 cycles every 3 weeks.	Every day for 5 years.	Treatment is for 12 months.
Side effects: fatigue, skin irritation, oedema, pain.	Side effects: D&V, mucocutaneous ulceration, hair loss, fatigue.	Side effects: hot flushes, affects bone density (tamoxifen ↑, AIs ↓ density).	Side effects: nausea, headaches, fatigue, cardiac complications.

- Is given post-operatively to all patients who undergo breast conservation surgery and reduces recurrence rates from ~35% to 10–12%.
- Post-mastectomy radiotherapy is required in ~20% of cases if the tumour is high grade, heavily node positive or in large or inflammatory cancers.
- Radiation is given every day for 3–5 weeks.
- Side effects include fatigue, local skin irritation, oedema and pain. There is ~1 in 1000 risk of radiation-induced cancer at 5–15 years.
- Chemotherapy.
  - Is given post-operatively to patients with aggressive tumours, in particular to patients with:
    - young age;
    - high tumour grade, node positive, or large primary cancer;
    - ER negative cancers;
    - HER-2 positive cancers;
    - triple negative cancers.
  - Side effects include mucocutaneous ulceration, nausea, vomiting, diarrhoea, hair loss and fatigue.
  - May be associated with more serious complications, such as neutropenic sepsis and bleeding as a result of bone marrow suppression.
  - May also result in infertility (from premature ovarian failure), increased risk of osteoporosis and cardiovascular disease.
  - Common agents include a combination of anthracyclines (e.g. doxorubicin), cyclophosphamides and taxanes.
- Adjuvant anti-oestrogen therapy.
  - ER receptor status is determined for all breast cancers and if positive, patients are treated with anti-oestrogen therapy.
  - Tamoxifen is used in pre-menopausal women for a period of 5 years.
    - It is a selective oestrogen receptor modulator and has an ER antagonist effect on breast cancer cells but an ER agonist effect on endometrial cells and bone.
    - Side effects include hot flushes, which are common, and a small increased risk of endometrial cancer from 1:100 000 to 2:100 000).
    - It has a bone density protective effect.
  - Aromatase inhibitors (e.g. Arimidex, Letrozole, Exemestane) are used in post-menopausal women, again for 5 years.
    - These drugs block the peripheral conversion of androgens to oestrogens, the main source of oestrogen in post-menopausal women. Oestrogen levels are thereby reduced to very low levels.
    - Side effects include hot flushes, joint pains and an increased risk of osteoporosis (bone density scans are required during therapy).

General surgery

- Adjuvant Anti-HER-2 directed therapy.
  - HER-2 (epidermal growth factor, EGFR-2) receptor is expressed in ⅓ of breast cancers and is a poor prognostic factor.
  - Trastuzumab (Herceptin®) is a monoclonal antibody that binds to HER-2 and reduces tumour growth.
  - Treatment with trastuzumab is for 12 months in patients with HER-2 positive tumours.

3.3.9 PROGNOSIS

- Prognosis for breast cancer is determined by several factors:
  - How aggressive the tumour is (indicated by tumour size, grade, receptor expression profile, presence of nodal disease and patient age).
  - The presence of distant metastases or inoperable disease at diagnosis. (Advanced disease is dealt with in more detail in Section 3.3.10).
- There are several prognostic tools now available to help calculate expected life expectancy. They also may aid patient understanding and can guide clinician decision making. They include:
  - the Nottingham Prognostic Index (NPI);
  - Adjuvant OnLine;
  - PREDICT.

> **MICRO-print**
> Calculating the NPI:
> NPI = tumour grade (1–3) + lymph node stage (1–3) + tumour size in cm × 0.2

3.3.10 ADVANCED BREAST CANCER

- Advanced breast cancer may refer to locally advanced or metastatic disease.
- Locally advanced disease (stage 3 in the TNM classification):
  - ulceration or invasion of skin;
  - tumours invading the chest wall;
  - tumours with a size greater than 5 cm;
  - palpable matted, inoperable lymph nodes.
- Inflammatory cancers are a special type of locally advanced breast cancer that are associated with a poorer prognosis.
  - They present as a warm, oedematous, erythematous breast that has an appearance similar to that of cellulitis.
    - Peau d'orange is a classic accompanying feature.
  - Inflammatory cancers are usually treated with primary chemotherapy followed by mastectomy and axillary node clearance.
- Metastatic breast cancer (stage 4 in the TNM classification):
  - 20–30% of all women with breast cancer will ultimately develop metastatic disease and die of their cancer.

- Metastatic disease is incurable but may be treated very effectively to prolong and enhance quality of life.
- Survival times are highly variable depending on the site of metastatic disease, disease burden and cancer biology.
  - A woman with low-volume, ER positive, bone metastases may survive for many years.
  - Survival for women with cerebral metastases is usually only a few months.
- Metastatic disease should be confirmed using appropriate imaging (e.g. CT, MRI, isotope bone scanning or PET scanning).

MICRO-facts

Common sites of breast cancer metastases include bone, lungs, brain and liver.

  - Biopsy confirmation is rarely required as imaging is usually pathognomonic.
- Management of metastatic disease includes hormone therapy, chemotherapy, radiotherapy, palliation of symptoms and social and psychological support.
  - Orthopaedic fixation of pathological fractures or pre-emptive stabilisation of severely weakened bones.
  - Anti-oestrogens.
  - Trastuzumab.
  - Radiation of painful bone secondaries.
  - Bisphosphonates for hypercalcaemia and bone pain.
  - Pleural drainage and pleurodesis for pleural effusions.
  - Blood transfusions for anaemia.
- In a woman presenting with metastatic disease at the time of diagnosis it is rarely appropriate to undertake surgical removal of the primary, as this has not been proven to enhance survival. Exceptions would be women whose primary disease is symptomatic.

MICRO-case

An 87-year-old woman presents to breast clinic with a large, ulcerating tumour on her left breast, associated with palpable, hard axillary lymph nodes. She undergoes triple assessment, which diagnoses an ER positive breast cancer with lymph node spread. The MDT recommended a staging CT scan that confirms the presence of liver and bone metastases. She is informed of the diagnosis and introduced to her breast care specialist nurse.

Learning points:
- A diagnosis of breast cancer is a life-changing event for most patients.
- Breast care nurses play a major role in the psychosocial support.

General surgery

3.4 BREAST SCREENING

- The NHS Breast Screening Programme (NHSBSP) started in 1987.
- Aims to detect breast cancer at a pre-clinical or early stage to optimize outcome.

3.4.1 EFFICACY OF BREAST SCREENING

- Leads to a 21% reduction in breast cancer-specific mortality in the 50–70 year age group.

3.4.2 WHAT SCREENING INVOLVES

- All women aged 50–70 are invited for mammography every 3 years.
  - This age range is being extended to include women aged 47–73 years over the next few years as part of a UK-wide randomised controlled trial.
- All images are double reported to improve sensitivity and specificity.
- Two radiological views are taken:
  - Cranio-caudal: Visualises more medial lesions.
  - Medio-lateral oblique: Visualises the lateral breast and axilla.
- 5% recall rate (decreases with increasing age).
- Further investigation consists of:
  - additional imaging (compression views/USS);
  - clinical breast examination;
  - biopsy (usually core biopsy).
- <66% will show no worrying changes after further investigation (see Figure 3.9).
- Between 6 and 8 women per 1000 screened will be diagnosed with cancer (see Figure 3.10).

3.4.3 RISKS OF BREAST SCREENING

- Recall for further investigation (including further imaging or biopsy).
- False positive diagnosis.
- False negative diagnosis.
- 'Radiation exposure' (negligible).
- Over-diagnosis of breast cancer (see MICRO-print box).
- Discomfort and anxiety.
- Interval cancers, i.e. cancers that are detected between screening visits.

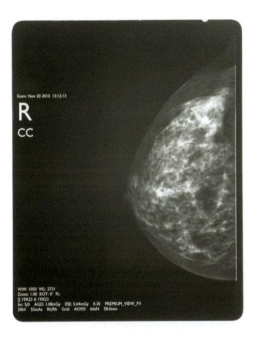

Figure 3.9 Normal mammogram. (From: *Obstetrics, Gynaecology, and Women's Health on the Move*, Figure 20.7a, p. 266.)

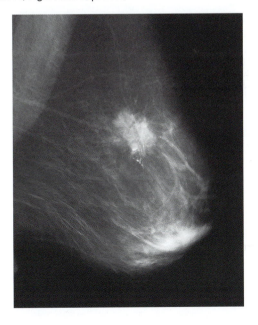

Figure 3.10 Spiculated mass—a breast cancer as seen on mammography. (From: *Obstetrics, Gynaecology, and Women's Health on the Move*, Figure 20.7b, p. 266.)

> **MICRO-print**
>
> Over-diagnosis:
> - Refers to the diagnosis of subclinical disease that would never have presented clinically within the patient's lifetime.
> - More relevant with increasing age due to competing causes of death and slower-growing cancers in older women.
> - Impossible to predict which lesions are going to become clinically important; therefore all lesions are acted on.

3.4.4 BENEFITS OF BREAST SCREENING

- Screening is more likely to detect cancers with a more favourable prognosis:
  - smaller cancers;
  - lower-grade cancers;
  - less likely to show lymphatic invasion;
  - less likely to involve axillary lymph nodes.
- More likely to be offered breast-conserving surgery vs. mastectomy.
- Less likely to require adjuvant chemotherapy.

> **MICRO-facts**
>
> Bias in screening programmes:
> - **Lead time bias:** Picking up of cancers through screening earlier than they would have presented clinically; therefore the patient appears to live longer with the disease (when all that has increased is the time of knowledge about the diagnosis).
> - **Length time bias:** Picking up of slower-growing, less aggressive cancers through screening; therefore again the patient appears to live longer.

4 Endocrine

4.1 EXAMINATION OF THE THYROID GLAND

- The thyroid gland is butterfly-shaped with two lobes connected by a central isthmus.
- It is located at the level of the second and third tracheal rings (Figure 4.1).
- A normal gland is palpable only in about 1/2 of women and 1/4 of men.
- Goitre = enlargement of the thyroid gland (see micro-facts box).

> ### MICRO-facts
>
> Goitre:
> - This term describes an enlargement of the thyroid, which can either be felt on examination or is visibly noticeable. There are many causes of a thyroid swelling and the patient may be hyper-, hypo- or euthyroid.
> - Causes:
>   - Physiological, occurring in pregnancy or at puberty (as thyroid hormones play a role in the pubertal growth spurt).
>   - Autoimmune disease (Graves' or Hashimoto's).
>   - Thyroiditis—There is diffuse swelling and this may be tender. It may occur in a viral illness and cause transient hyperthyroidism.
>   - Iodine deficiency (also known as Derbyshire neck).
>   - Toxic multi-nodular goitre. A nodular goitre can also occur due to thyroid cysts or fibrosis.
>   - Thyroid tumours may cause an isolated, unilateral swelling. Malignancy should be suspected in any solitary thyroid nodule; however most are benign.
>   - Others—e.g., TB, sarcoidosis.

4.1.1 EXAMINATION SEQUENCE

Inspection

- Standing in front of the patient, look for any obvious thyroid swellings or asymmetry.
- Stridor may also be present if there is airway compression.
- Provide the patient with a glass of water and inspect again whilst they

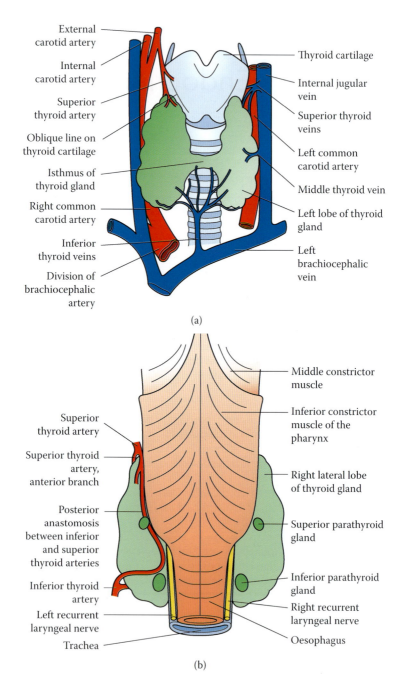

Figure 4.1 Thyroid gland and its relations: (a) anterior view and (b) posterior view. (From: *Illustrated Clinical Anatomy, 2nd Edition*, Figure 22.7, p. 350.)

swallow a sip. The thyroid moves upwards on swallowing, as it is contained within the pretracheal fascia, which is attached to the cricoid cartilage.

Palpation

- With the patient sitting relaxed, stand behind him or her and place your hands on the front of his or her neck with your fingertips just touching (Figure 4.2).
- Remember to be gentle when doing this, as it can be quite uncomfortable for patients. Be alert for any signs of distress.
- Ask the patient to swallow again whilst your hands are in position over the gland. Note the size, shape and consistency of any goitre or nodule, and the presence or absence of a thrill.
  - In Graves' disease, a goitre is usually smooth and diffuse, whereas it is irregular in a multi-nodular goitre.
  - Most goitres will move upwards on swallowing; however invasive cancer may fix the gland to adjacent structures.

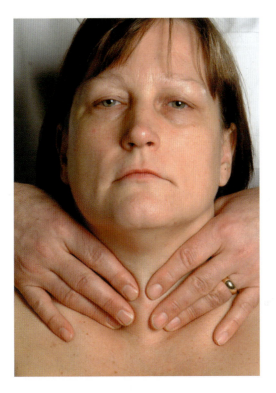

Figure 4.2 Palpate the thyroid gland from behind. (From: *Browse's Introduction to the Symptoms and Signs of Surgical Disease, 4th Edition*, Figure 11.33, p. 291.)

- When assessing thyroid nodules, note if they are single or multiple, large or small. A hard nodule is more suggestive of malignancy.
- Note whether the gland is tender; diffuse tenderness suggests viral thyroiditis.

Auscultation

- Using the diaphragm of your stethoscope, listen over the gland for any bruit. If present, a bruit indicates abnormally high blood flow as in hyperthyroidism, and may be associated with a palpable thrill.

4.2 HYPERTHYROIDISM

- Synonymous with 'overactive thyroid' and 'thyrotoxicosis'. See Figure 4.3.

4.2.1 EPIDEMIOLOGY

- Incidence of 0.2–0.3% of men and 2–3% women.

4.2.2 AETIOLOGY

Graves' disease (autoimmune)

- Occurs in females, aged 20–40.

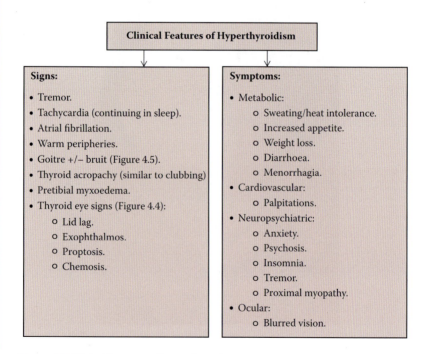

Signs:	Symptoms:
• Tremor.	• Metabolic:
• Tachycardia (continuing in sleep).	o Sweating/heat intolerance.
• Atrial fibrillation.	o Increased appetite.
• Warm peripheries.	o Weight loss.
• Goitre +/– bruit (Figure 4.5).	o Diarrhoea.
• Thyroid acropachy (similar to clubbing)	o Menorrhagia.
• Pretibial myxoedema.	• Cardiovascular:
• Thyroid eye signs (Figure 4.4):	o Palpitations.
o Lid lag.	• Neuropsychiatric:
o Exophthalmos.	o Anxiety.
o Proptosis.	o Psychosis.
o Chemosis.	o Insomnia.
	o Tremor.
	o Proximal myopathy.
	• Ocular:
	o Blurred vision.

Clinical Features of Hyperthyroidism

Figure 4.3 Clinical features of hyperthyroidism.

General surgery

- The body produces antibodies that are structurally similar to the binding site of TSH, causing excessive release of T3 and T4 by the thyroid.
- There is an association with other autoimmune conditions (e.g., type I diabetes mellitus, vitiligo, Addison's disease).
- May occur following infection with *Yersinia* or *E. coli*.
- Eye signs (exophthalmos, lid lag) are more common in Graves' disease (Figure 4.4).
- May have a smooth, enlarged thyroid gland.

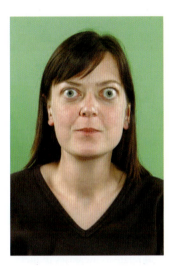

Figure 4.4 Eye signs in Graves' disease. (From: *Bailey & Love's Short Practice of Surgery, 26th Edition*, Figure 51.25, p. 755.)

MICRO-facts

Hyperthyroidism is usually due to an inherent thyroid abnormality; pituitary causes are rare.

Toxic multi-nodular goitre

- Occurs in older women.
- Areas of hyper- and hypoplasia within the gland.
- Palpable nodular goitre (Figure 4.5).

Toxic adenoma

- Causes ~5% of hyperthyroidism.
- Will not remit after anti-thyroid medication.

General surgery

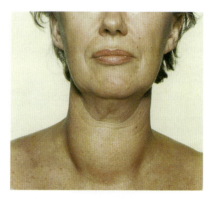

Figure 4.5 A large colloid goitre. (From: *Bailey & Love's Short Practice of Surgery, 25th Edition*, Figure 11.36, p. 296.)

- Focal point of enlargement palpable within the gland.
- Post-partum thyroiditis.
- De Quervain's thyroiditis (following acute inflammation).
- Testicular or ovarian tumours.
- Pituitary adenoma.
- Overdose of thyroxine.

4.2.3 CLINICAL FEATURES

- Features are systemic and relate to increases in metabolism and energy consumption (see Figure 4.3).

4.2.4 DIAGNOSIS

- Hyperthyroidism is confirmed by thyroid function tests (TFTs):
    - ↓TSH (<0.5 mU/L);
    - ↑T3 and T4 (except in rare pituitary or gonadal causes).
- In Graves' disease, thyroid peroxidase (TPO) and thyroglobulin antibodies can be measured.

Imaging

- Thyroid scintogram uses radioactive iodine to identify overactive areas within the gland ('hot nodules').
- Ultrasound scan (USS) and computed tomography (CT) allow detail of the gland and identification of compression of adjacent structures.

Biopsy

- Allows histological analysis.
- Often USS-guided.

4.2.5 TREATMENT

Medication

- Anti-thyroid drugs can be used definitively or in preparation for surgery.
  - Carbimazole (first line) or propylthiouracil.
    - Acts by interfering with hormone synthesis.
- 'Block and replace' (high-dose anti-thyroid drugs to completely suppress hormone production alongside replacement thyroxine) or suppression with lower doses, aiming for lower hormone levels.
- Complication of carbimazole therapy:
  - Agranulocytosis (severe bone marrow suppression); therefore any infections must be thoroughly investigated during treatment.
- Control of symptoms, such as palpitations and tremor, may be provided by beta-blockade with propranolol.
- Achieves control in ~50% after 1 year of treatment.

Radio-iodine

- As the thyroid is the only organ to take up iodine, radioactive isotopes (I^{131}) can be given to destroy the thyroid gland.
- It is contra-indicated in children and pregnancy.

Surgery

- May be partial or total excision depending on the cause.
  - In a subtotal thyroidectomy the posterior rim is left so to avoid damage to the parathyroid glands.
- Four main indications for surgery over medical therapy:
  - when a quick, effective treatment is desired (e.g. in young women with Graves' disease);
  - when anti-thyroid drugs have proved ineffective;
  - toxic multi-nodular goitre (better medical and cosmetic outcome);
  - toxic solitary nodule (often resistant to medical treatment).
- Pre-operative considerations:
  - Thyroid function should be normalised as much as possible to avoid the dangers of thyrotoxicosis and thyroid storm.
  - Anti-thyroid drugs are often stopped 10–14 days pre-operatively as they increase vascularity to the gland.
- Complications:
  - Hypothyroidism occurs in ~10% at 1 year and increases with time.
  - Transient hypocalcaemia occurs ~10%, or permanently in ~1%. It is due to inadvertent damage to, or removal of, the parathyroid glands.
  - Hyperthyroidism—Late recurrence due to inadequate excision.
  - Thyroid crisis (rare). May occur in any hyperthyroid patient due to infection, surgery or stress.

General surgery

- There is hyperpyrexia, tachycardia and mania. It may cause death due to heart failure.
  - Treatment is with urgent propranolol, potassium iodide, anti-thyroid drugs and corticosteroids, along with supportive measures.
- Recurrent laryngeal nerve injury occurs in 2–3%. May cause slight 'hoarseness' of voice to complete loss of vocal function and critical airway narrowing. Damage to the external nerve will cause a change in the quality of the voice.
- Tracheal damage or pneumothorax may occur acutely due to direct surgical damage or due to tracheomalacia, following many years of tracheal compression from a goitre.
- Haemorrhage—A potential complication of any surgery; in the neck this is an emergency, as it may cause tracheal compression. The wound is usually stitched with one continuous suture that may be pulled out in one go if there is life-threatening compression.

4.2.6 PROGNOSIS

- Slight increase in mortality in the first year following diagnosis of hyperthyroidism; the reason for this is unknown.
- Adequately treated hyperthyroidism results in an increased risk of osteoporosis.

MICRO-case

A 32-year-old woman presents with a fluttering feeling in her chest. She also complains of 'looking funny'. On further questioning she has been suffering from diarrhoea recently. On examination she is wearing a t-shirt (despite the cold, wintery weather) and is sweating. She has a fine tremor and her eyes appear to be protruding. You also note that she is in fast atrial fibrillation.

TFTs reveal a ↓ TSH in association with ↑ T3 and ↑ T4. Further tests reveal positive thyroid receptor antibodies, and a 'hot' thyroid nodule is demonstrated on radio-isotope scanning. She is diagnosed with Graves' disease and treated with carbimazole in combination with a beta-blocker to control her heart rate.

Learning points:

- 75% of patients with Graves' disease have associated eye signs.
- Presentation can be very vague.
- She should be warned about the risks of agranulocytosis with carbimazole.
- There is a high risk of relapse so surgical excision may be required.

4.3 HYPOTHYROIDISM

4.3.1 EPIDEMIOLOGY

- Lifetime prevalence of 9.3% in women and 1.3% in men.

4.3.2 AETIOLOGY

Congenital

- Agenesis or maldescent of the gland.

Defects in hormone synthesis

- Iodine deficiency (commonest cause worldwide, rare in the UK).
- Dyshormonogenesis (e.g. Pendred's syndrome)—rare and often familial.
- Over-treatment of hyperthyroidism.

Autoimmune

- Most common cause.
- Antibodies causing inflammation and fibrosis of the gland resulting in atrophy (atrophic thyroiditis) or increase in size (Hashimoto's thyroiditis).
- May be associated with other autoimmune conditions.
- Following thyroid surgery.
- Infective.

Secondary

- Hypopituitarism.
- Peripheral resistance to thyroid hormone.

4.3.3 CLINICAL FEATURES

- Often the opposite to hyperthyroidism and reflects a reduction in basal metabolic rate and reduced energy consumption (see Figure 4.6).

4.3.4 DIAGNOSIS

Biochemistry

- Primary hypothyroidism is confirmed by $\uparrow$ TSH with an associated $\downarrow$ T4.
- Other abnormalities associated with a hypothyroid state include:
  - anaemia;
  - raised AST (from the liver or muscle);
  - raised creatinine kinase;
  - hypercholesterolaemia;
  - hyponatraemia (due to increased ADH);
  - hyperprolactinaemia.

General surgery

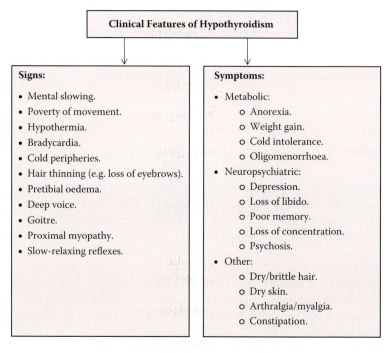

Clinical Features of Hypothyroidism

Signs:

- Mental slowing.
- Poverty of movement.
- Hypothermia.
- Bradycardia.
- Cold peripheries.
- Hair thinning (e.g. loss of eyebrows).
- Pretibial oedema.
- Deep voice.
- Goitre.
- Proximal myopathy.
- Slow-relaxing reflexes.

Symptoms:

- Metabolic:
    o Anorexia.
    o Weight gain.
    o Cold intolerance.
    o Oligomenorrhoea.
- Neuropsychiatric:
    o Depression.
    o Loss of libido.
    o Poor memory.
    o Loss of concentration.
    o Psychosis.
- Other:
    o Dry/brittle hair.
    o Dry skin.
    o Arthralgia/myalgia.
    o Constipation.

Figure 4.6 Clinical features of hyperthyroidism.

- Anti-thyroid antibodies in Hashimoto's thyroiditis:
    - anti-thyroglobulin;
    - anti-mitochondrial antibodies.
- Imaging:
    - As for imaging of a goitre in hyperthyroidism (see Section 4.3.4).

4.3.5 TREATMENT

- Thyroxine replacement for life.
    - Started slowly and titrated carefully to avoid cardiac complications.
    - Adequate replacement should be achieved within 6 weeks and confirmed on biochemical testing.
- Surgery is not usually required in hypothyroidism but may be indicated in Hashimoto's thyroiditis if there is a large goitre causing compression symptoms.

4.4 CARCINOMA OF THE THYROID GLAND

4.4.1 AETIOLOGY

- Rare, primary thyroid cancer accounts for ~0.5% of all malignancies.
- M:F ratio 1:2.

- Often arises in pre-existing goitres.
- Associations with exposure to ionising radiation in childhood.

4.4.2 CLINICAL FEATURES

- Usually presents as a solitary nodule or as part of a multi-nodular goitre.

> ## MICRO-facts
> Suspicious features in a patient with a goitre:
> - Hoarse voice.
> - A hard nodule.
> - Lymphadenopathy.

4.4.3 DIAGNOSIS

- Ultrasound scans can detect solid nodules.
- Most thyroid swellings can be diagnosed with FNAC (the exception is follicular cancer).
- X-rays: Chest x-ray (CXR) to diagnose metastases. Skeletal x-rays in presence of bone pain.
- Calcitonin levels if medullary carcinoma is suspected.
- Seek evidence of MEN-2 syndrome if medullary cancer is diagnosed.

4.4.4 PATHOLOGY

- There are four discrete types of primary thyroid cancer (Table 4.1):

> ## MICRO-print
> Thyroid lymphomas and metastases from breast, lung, kidney and prostate are rare but do occur.

- papillary;
- follicular;
- medullary;
- anaplastic.

> ## MICRO-facts
> **Calcium haemostasis is very important.**
>
> Decreased serum calcium leads to neural excitability and eventually tetany. Hypercalcaemia can cause hypertension, cardiac arrhythmias and left ventricular hypertrophy. It may also cause hypercalcaemic crisis: drowsiness, confusion, coma, dehydration, weakness, vomiting and renal failure.

General surgery

Table 4.1 Classification of thyroid cancers.

	PAPILLARY	FOLLICULAR	MEDULLARY	ANAPLASTIC
Incidence	60%	20%	5–8%	5%
Age	Any age with peak incidence 3rd/4th decades.	Middle age, peak incidence 5th decade.	May occur at any age.	Occurs in the elderly.
Pathology	Slow-growing, often multicentric. Pale, empty-looking 'orphan Annie' nuclei. TSH dependent.	Usually unifocal. Difficult to differentiate benign from malignant on FNAC alone.	Arises from parafollicular C cells, secretes calcitonin. Can be multifocal.	Rapidly growing and locally invasive. Undifferentiated.
Metastatic spread	Metastasises early to local nodes.	Haematogenous spread to lung and bone.	May spread to cervical nodes.	Early spread via lymphatics and blood to lungs, bone and brain.
Treatment	Total lobectomy or thyroidectomy. Thyroxine for life.	Total lobectomy or thyroidectomy. Thyroxine for life.	Total thyroidectomy and routine neck dissection.	Debulking surgery and palliative radiotherapy. Tracheal stents may be needed.
Prognosis	90% 10-year survival.	>80% in small tumours.	>80% in small tumours. Associated with MEN-2.	90% die within 1 year (average survival 6–8 months).

4.5 PRIMARY HYPERPARATHYROIDISM

- The parathyroid glands are involved in calcium haemostasis (see Figure 4.7).

4.5.1 AETIOLOGY

- 85% due to a parathyroid adenoma.
- 15% due to diffuse parathyroid hyperplasia.
- Carcinoma of the parathyroid glands is rare.

4.5.2 CLINICAL FEATURES

Renal

- Renal or ureteric stones (most common clinical manifestation).
- UTI associated with calculi.

Skeletal

- Spontaneous fractures.
- Bone pain.
- Deformed, decalcified bones with cyst formation: osteitis fibrosa cystica.

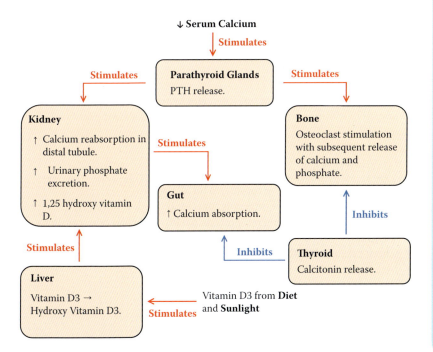

Figure 4.7 Calcium haemostasis.

Abdominal pain

- Constipation is common.
- Dyspepsia or frank duodenal ulceration.
- Pancreatitis.

> ## MICRO-facts
>
> Remember clinical features of hyperparathyroidism are features of raised calcium: **stones**, **bones**, **abdominal groans**, and **psychic moans**.

Psychiatric manifestations

- Depression.
- Psychosis.
- Confusion.

Other

- Thirst.
- Polyuria.
- Muscle weakness.
- Fatigue.

4.5.3 DIAGNOSIS

- Raised parathyroid hormone (PTH).
- Elevated serum calcium.
- Low serum phosphate.
- Assess renal function to rule out secondary hyperparathyroidism.
- Sestamibi scanning will identify a solitary adenoma, allowing selective removal.

4.5.4 TREATMENT

- Surgical excision should be considered for all patients.
- Cinacalcet may be used if surgery is contra-indicated. It works by binding to calcium-sensing receptors on parathyroid chief cells, causing a ↓ PTH.
- Check calcium daily in the post-operative period to avoid hypocalcaemia.
- May require calcium and vitamin D supplements.

4.5.5 SECONDARY HYPERPARATHYROIDISM

- 10% of all hyperparathyroidism.
- Due to hyperplasia of all four glands secondary to low persistent serum calcium.

- Usually occurs in patients with chronic renal failure due to several reasons:
  - ↑ serum phosphate stimulates PTH (even if serum calcium is normal).
  - Failure to synthesise vitamin D.
  - ↓ calcium, which stimulates PTH production directly.
- Treatment includes correcting the underlying cause. May still require surgical excision of glands with long-term calcium supplements.

4.5.6 TERTIARY HYPERPARATHYROIDISM

- Prolonged secondary hyperparathyroidism results in autonomous PTH production, which continues even after removal of the stimulus (i.e. following renal transplant in chronic renal failure patients).

4.6 PHAEOCHROMOCYTOMA

4.6.1 AETIOLOGY

- Rare neuroendocrine tumour of chromaffin cells of (usually) the adrenal medulla.
- Catecholamine-secreting tumour cells (adrenaline, noradrenaline, dopamine).
- May also secrete vasopressin, somatostatin, ACTH and oxytocin.

> **MICRO-facts**
>
> Phaeochromocytomas approximately follow the rule of 10%:
> - 10% are malignant.
> - 10% are bilateral.
> - 10% are familial.
> - 10% are extra-adrenal.

4.6.2 CLINICAL FEATURES

- Signs and symptoms are those of sympathetic nervous system hyperactivity, e.g.:
  - paroxysmal hypertension;
  - tachycardia;
  - palpitations;
  - tremor;
  - sweating;
  - anxiety.

4.6.3 INVESTIGATIONS

- 24-hour urine for metanephrines and catecholamines (vanillylmandelic acid).
- Raised plasma catecholamine levels.
- Abdominal CT/MRI (magnetic resonance imaging) to demonstrate tumour.
- Meta-iodobenzylguanidine (MIBG) scan—radioisotope scan.

4.6.4 MANAGEMENT

- Resection of tumour, preferably laparoscopically.
- Pre-operative control of hypertension as tumour manipulation will result in catecholamine release.
- α-Blockade with phenoxybenzamine prior to β-blockade with propranolol.

4.6.5 PROGNOSIS

- 95% 5-year survival if not malignant (i.e. 90% of tumours).

4.7 CONN'S SYNDROME (PRIMARY HYPERALDOSTERONISM)

4.7.1 AETIOLOGY

- Rare aldosterone-secreting tumour (benign or malignant) of the adrenal cortex.

4.7.2 CLINICAL FEATURES

- Usually asymptomatic.
- Headaches.
- Hypertension.
- Features of hypokalaemia.

> **MICRO-facts**
>
> Features of hypokalaemia:
> - Muscle weakness.
> - Tetany.
> - Polydipsia.
> - Polyuria.

4.7.3 INVESTIGATIONS

- Increased plasma aldosterone levels.
- U&Es: raised sodium, low potassium.
- CT scan to visualise tumour.

4.7.4 MANAGEMENT

- Laparoscopic adrenalectomy.
- Pre-operative spironolactone for 4 weeks to correct hypokalaemia.

4.8 CUSHING'S SYNDROME

4.8.1 EPIDEMIOLOGY

- Usually occurs in young adults.
- M:F ratio M < F.

4.8.2 AETIOLOGY

- Increased levels of circulating cortisol.
- Commonest cause is exogenous administration of steroids.

Primary adrenal disease
- Adrenal adenoma.
- Adrenal carcinoma.

Secondary adrenal disease
- ACTH-secreting pituitary adenoma (Cushing's disease).
- ACTH-secreting tumour, e.g. oat-cell carcinoma of the lung.

4.8.3 CLINICAL FEATURES

- See Figure 4.8.

4.8.4 INVESTIGATIONS

- Increased levels of plasma cortisol.
  - Loss of diurnal variation of plasma cortisol.
  - Increase 24-hour urinary cortisol levels.
  - Inappropriately high night-time salivary cortisol.
    - 11 p.m. salivary cortisol is the gold standard screening test.
- Dexamethasone suppression test:
  - Dexamethasone suppresses pituitary ACTH secretion.
  - Administered over 48 hours and plasma cortisol is measured.
  - In normal individuals, negative feedback results in ↓ ACTH and cortisol.

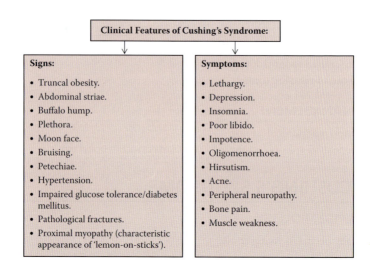

Figure 4.8 Clinical features of Cushing's syndrome.

MICRO-facts

Cushing's **syndrome** is an excess of circulating glucocorticoids.
Cushing's **disease** is when this increase is due to a pituitary tumour.

4.8.5 MANAGEMENT

- Stop exogenous steroid excess if this is the cause.
- Laparoscopic adrenalectomy if adrenal adenoma.
  - Will require lifelong steroid replacement if bilateral.
- Trans-sphenoidal hypophysectomy if pituitary adenoma.

4.9 MULTIPLE ENDOCRINE NEOPLASIA (MEN)

4.9.1 DEFINITION

- Rare, autosomal dominant, inherited syndrome of endocrine tumours.

4.9.2 CLASSIFICATION

- MEN is classified as type 1, type 2A and type 2B (see Table 4.2).

4.9.3 INVESTIGATIONS

- Genetic screening for offspring of known sufferers.
- Relevant tests for specific tumours.

Table 4.2 Classification of the MEN syndromes.

	MEN-1	MEN-2A	MEN-2B
Gene	Tumour suppressor gene on chromosome 11 encoding for the protein menin.	Mutation of RET proto-oncogene on chromosome 10 encoding for a transmembrane glycoprotein receptor.	Mutation of RET proto-oncogene on chromosome 10 encoding for a transmembrane glycoprotein receptor.
Tumours	Parathyroid. Pancreatic, e.g. gastrinoma or insulinoma. Pituitary, e.g. prolactinoma. Adrenocortical.	Medullary carcinoma of the thyroid. Phaeochromocytoma. Parathyroid.	Medullary carcinoma of the thyroid. Phaeochromocytoma. Neuromas of lips, tongue, cheeks and eyelids.
Other information			Marfanoid appearance. Visceral ganglioneuromas.

4.9.4 MANAGEMENT

- Surgical resection of tumours.
- Dopamine agonists, e.g. bromocriptine for prolactinomas.

Hepatobiliary

5.1 HEPATOBILIARY ANATOMY

- Biliary and pancreatic relations are shown in Figures 5.1 and 5.2.

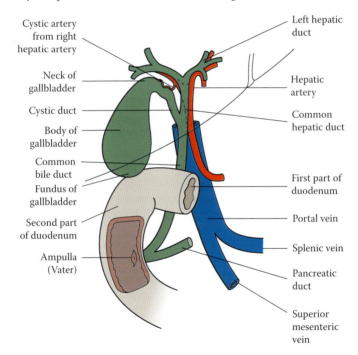

Cystic artery from right hepatic artery

Neck of gallbladder

Cystic duct

Body of gallbladder

Common bile duct

Fundus of gallbladder

Second part of duodenum

Ampulla (Vater)

Left hepatic duct

Hepatic artery

Common hepatic duct

First part of duodenum

Portal vein

Splenic vein

Pancreatic duct

Superior mesenteric vein

Figure 5.1 Biliary anatomy. (From: *Illustrated Clinical Anatomy*, Figure 7.9, p. 104.)

5.2 UPPER ABDOMINAL PAIN

5.2.1 HISTORY

- A careful history is essential to identify the likely cause of the pain:
    - Colicky pain—suggests pathology of a hollow viscus.
    - Constant pain—suggests an inflammatory or malignant cause.

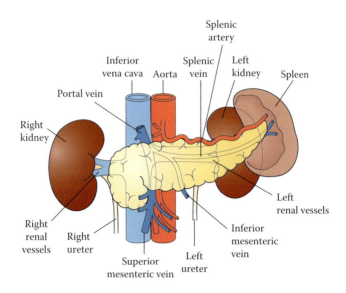

Figure 5.2 Relations of the pancreas posteriorly. (From: *Bailey & Love's Short Practice of Surgery, 26th Edition*, Figure 68.1, p. 1118.)

- Severe pain—if out of proportion to findings, suggests ischaemia.
- Pain radiating through to the back—suggestive of a retroperitoneal organ, e.g. pancreas, kidney, aorta.
- It is important to note the location, onset, character and timing of the pain, as well as any associated symptoms (Figure 5.3, Table 5.1).

5.2.2 EXAMINATION

- Patients should be examined according to the examination sequence below (Section 5.3).

5.2.3 INVESTIGATIONS

FBC

- ↑ white cell count (WCC) in infection or inflammation.
- Microcytic anaemia may indicate iron deficiency caused by chronic blood loss (gastritis, oesophagitis, malignancy).
  - Note: In acute severe bleeding, the haemoglobin level may be normal, as there may not have been time for fluid redistribution. **Do not be falsely reassured.**
- Macrocytic anaemia may be due to B_{12} deficiency, which is associated with atrophic gastritis or high alcohol consumption, which may be linked to cirrhosis and pancreatitis.
- Raised platelets may be caused by haemorrhage.

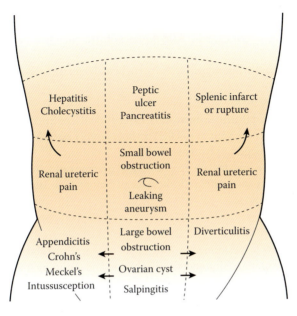

Figure 5.3 Regions of the abdomen in which pain is experienced. (From: *Browse's Introduction to the Investigation and Management of Surgical Disease*, Figure 17.1, p. 373.)

Table 5.1 Causes of acute and chronic abdominal pain.

REGION OF ABDOMEN	ACUTE PAIN	CHRONIC PAIN
Right hypochondrium	Pneumonia. Pulmonary embolism. Cholecystitis. Ascending cholangitis. Biliary colic. Hepatitis. Hepatic abscess.	Empyema of gallbladder. Hepatitis. Hepatic abscess. Hepatomegaly of any cause. Hepatic flexure tumour.
Epigastrium	Myocardial infarction. Oesophagitis. Gastritis. Peptic ulcer. Peptic colic. Pancreatitis.	Oesophagitis. Gastritis. Gastric tumour. Peptic ulcer. Pancreatitis. Pancreatic tumour.
Left hypochondrium	Pneumonia. Pulmonary embolism. Splenic infarction/rupture. Pancreatitis.	Pancreatitis. Splenomegaly. Splenic flexure tumour. Ischaemic stricture.

General surgery

Liver function test (LFT)

- ↑ conjugated bilirubin and ↑ ALP if stones obstructing the common bile duct.
- Raised transaminases suggest liver parenchymal damage such as hepatitis.

Serum amylase levels

- May be elevated in acute pancreatitis. Over 1000 iU, or five times the upper reference limit of in your hospital, is pathognomic. Lesser degrees of elevation are suggestive but not diagnostic.
  - Note: Serum amylase may be normal in some cases, such as acute on chronic pancreatitis and where the patient presents late in the course of the disease.

Chest radiograph

- Should always be performed in acute upper or generalised abdominal pain to rule out perforation (air under the diaphragm and outlining the falciform ligament).
- If pneumonia is suspected.

Abdominal radiograph

- Indicated in cases where bowel obstruction is clinically suspected but is otherwise not usually useful.
- May show calcification of gallstones or chronic pancreatitis.
- There may be ground glass sign in pancreatitis.
- May also show free air (Rigler's sign) in perforation.

Ultrasound scan

- May identify numerous pathologies, e.g. gallstones, abscess, biliary obstruction, metastatic disease, splenomegaly, splenic rupture, AAA.

Endoscopy

- In suspected gastritis, peptic ulcer disease or gastro-oesophageal malignancy.

CT scan

- Good if unsure about diagnosis, as will show pathology in solid organs.
- Use only if indicated, as involves a higher dose of radiation than plain x-rays and is more expensive than ultrasound (US).

Magnetic resonance imaging and MR cholangiopancreatography (MRCP)

- Is used in a diagnostic capacity in biliary obstruction.
- If chronic pancreatitis or pancreatic malignancy suspected.

General surgery

- Resolving diagnosis of liver lesions:
    - MR is the gold standard assessment to differentiate haemangiomas and metastases, fatty liver, etc. and in assessing extent of liver malignancy prior to surgery.

Endoscopic retrograde cholangiopancreatography (ERCP)

- Is used in both a diagnostic (although this is being replaced with MRCP) and therapeutic capacity in biliary obstruction or pancreatobiliary malignancy.
- Can be used to relieve biliary obstruction associated with pancreatitis.

Electrocardiogram (ECG)

- If MI suspected.

MICRO-facts

Remember the 4 Cs in GI causes of clubbing:
- **C**oeliac disease.
- **C**rohn's disease.
- Ulcerative **c**olitis.
- **C**irrhosis (hepatic or biliary).

5.3 HOW TO EXAMINE THE ABDOMEN

- Wash your hands.
- Introduce yourself and confirm the patient's identity.
- With the patient supine, expose the patient from just below the breasts to the groin. Keep the genitalia covered until these are specifically examined to maintain patient dignity.

5.3.1 GENERAL INSPECTION

- Look at body mass (obese or signs of weight loss).
- Is the patient distressed?
- What is his or her colour (is there jaundice or pallor)?
- Look for clues around the bed, e.g. commode, drain tubes, catheters, drips or medications.

5.3.2 INSPECTION OF THE HANDS

- Look for the following:
    - finger clubbing;
    - palmar erythema (a sign of chronic liver disease);
    - pallor of the palmar creases (a sign of anaemia);
    - leuconychia (white nail beds; seen in hypoalbuminaemia);
    - koilonychia (spoon-shaped nails; seen in iron deficiency anaemia);
    - Dupuytren's contracture (fibromatosis of the palmar fascia).

General surgery

5.3.3 EXAMINATION OF THE ARMS

- Look for scratch marks (hyperbilirubinaemia causes pruritis).
- Assess for a liver flap (seen in liver failure) by asking the patient to dorsiflex his or her wrists for 15 seconds.
- Feel the pulse for tachycardia (a sign of sepsis or hypovolaemia).
- Check the blood pressure (may be low, indicating hypovolaemia or septic shock).

5.3.4 INSPECTION OF THE FACE

- Look at the eyes for:
  - jaundice (seen in the sclera);
  - pale conjunctiva (a sign of anaemia);
  - Kayser-Fleischer rings (a sign of Wilson's disease);
  - xanthelasmata (can be a sign of primary biliary cirrhosis).
- Look at the mouth for:
  - angular stomatitis (can be a sign of iron deficiency anaemia);
  - glossitis (can be a sign of iron, folate or B_{12} deficiency);
  - leukoplakia on the tongue (a white premalignant lesion);
  - telangiectasia;
  - aphthous ulcers (can be a sign of Crohn's disease);
  - fetor hepaticus (sweet-smelling breath seen in liver disease).

MICRO-facts

5 Fs of abdominal distension:
- **F**at.
- **F**luid.
- **F**aeces.
- **F**latus.
- **F**oetus.

5.3.5 EXAMINATION OF THE CHEST AND NECK

- Examine for supraclavicular lymphadenopathy.
- Are there any spider naevi (central arteriole with radiating dilated vessels seen with increased circulating oestrogens secondary to liver disease)?
- In males, is there gynaecomastia (indicating high oestrogen levels secondary to liver disease)?

MICRO-facts

A palpable **left** supraclavicular fossa lymph node (Virchow's node) can indicate gastric malignancy: Troisier's sign.

General surgery

5.3.6 INSPECTION OF THE ABDOMEN

- Look for:
  - scars;
  - abdominal distension;
  - any masses;
  - caput medusae (dilated periumbilical venous plexus seen in portal hypertension);
  - visible pulsation (indicating an AAA);
  - visible peristalsis (may indicate small bowel obstruction).

5.3.7 PALPATION OF THE ABDOMEN

- Having first asked the patient if they have any painful or tender areas in the abdomen, you should now palpate the abdomen.
- Keeping your hand flat, palpate the nine regions of the abdomen (see Figure 5.3).
- Assess gently for tenderness, watching the patient's face for signs of discomfort.
- Assess the size, shape, consistency, pulsatility and tenderness of any masses.
- Palpate for hepatomegaly. Moving from the right lower quadrant to the right costal margin, gently press inward and upward during the inspiratory phase of respiration to detect the liver edge as it descends on inspiration.
- Palpate for splenomegaly the same way, moving from the right lower quadrant toward the left upper quadrant. Ask the patient to roll toward you as you near the left costal margin and gently lift the left lower ribs forward to maximise your chances of feeling the spleen.
- Palpate for renal masses by placing one hand in the renal angle posteriorly and the other on the flank region anteriorly and gently pull the posterior hand forward to move any renal mass toward your other hand (balloting).
- Palpate for an enlarged bladder starting at the umbilicus and working down to the pubic symphysis. Ask if the patient needs to void before doing so to avoid discomfort.
- If pyloric obstruction is suspected, test for a succussion splash (sloshing heard on moving the stomach from side to side).
- Examine for aortic pulsation (expansile pulsation is felt if an AAA is present).
- Examine for inguinal lymphadenopathy.
- Examine the hernia orifices (see Section 2.2).
- Percussion:
  - Ascites sounds dull to percussion and will demonstrate shifting dullness (the dull area will become resonant with the patient rolled on his or her side as the fluid redistributes due to gravity).
  - Percuss for hepatomegaly (a change from a resonant to a dull note indicates the liver margins).

General surgery

- Percuss for splenomegaly in the same way.
- Percuss for bladder distension, progressively down from the umbilicus. Again, ask if the patient needs to void before doing so to avoid discomfort.
- Auscultation for bowel sounds:
  - Are they present? (If absent for >2 minutes this indicates a paralytic ileus).
  - Are they high-pitched and tinkling? (Can be a sign of bowel obstruction).
- The following steps must be performed with a chaperone present and after full explanation and verbal consent.
  - Perform a digital rectal examination.
  - Examination of the external genitalia in the male (see Section 9.1).
  - In all cases of lower abdominal pain in the female (e.g. suspected pelvic inflammatory disease, pelvic appendicitis), a gynaecological pelvic examination is also required unless the patient is 'virgo intacta'.

5.4 JAUNDICE: PATHOPHYSIOLOGY AND CLASSIFICATION

- Jaundice is the elevation of serum bilirubin (>9 mmol/L) and is clinically detectable at ~40 mmol/L or above.
- Bilirubin is the main breakdown product of haemoglobin and is found in the plasma in its unconjugated form bound to albumin. In the liver, it is conjugated with glucuronic acid prior to excretion in the bile.
- It is possible to determine the cause of jaundice depending on whether it is predominantly present in its conjugated or unconjugated form.
  - Raised unconjugated bilirubin indicates a pre-hepatic cause such as increased haemolysis (see Table 5.2).
  - Predominantly raised conjugated bilirubin indicates a hepatic or post-hepatic (obstructive) cause (see Table 5.2).
- Determining whether jaundice is pre-hepatic, hepatic or post-hepatic is also aided by other LFT results (Figure 5.4).
  - In pre-hepatic causes other LFTs are usually normal.
  - In hepatic, the transaminases are usually very high relative to the ALP.
  - In post-hepatic, the ALP is very high relative to the transaminases.

General surgery

Table 5.2 Features of pre-hepatic, hepatic and post-hepatic jaundice.

	PRE-HEPATIC	HEPATIC	POST-HEPATIC
Causes	**Increased breakdown of red blood cells:** Spherocytosis. Autoimmune. Haemolytic anaemia. Incompatible blood transfusion. Resorption of haematoma. Sickle cell disease. Hypersplenism.	**Decreased conjugation:** Cirrhosis. Hepatitis. Drug/toxin reactions. Crigler-Najjer syndrome. Gilbert syndrome. Dubin-Johnson syndrome. **Decreased hepatocyte uptake:** Sepsis. Drug/toxin reaction. **Liver tumours:** Primary and secondary.	**Bile duct obstruction:** Gallstones. Biliary stricture. Tumour: cholangiocarcinoma, ampullary or pancreatic. **Canaliculi obstruction:** Inflammatory swelling of hepatocytes (hepatitis/cirrhosis). Cholestasis (pregnancy, drug reaction).
Jaundice	Unconjugated. Mild jaundice, bilirubin rarely >100 mmol/L.	May be conjugated or unconjugated. Variable jaundice.	Conjugated. Variable jaundice, bilirubin may reach >1000 mmol/L.
Urine	Normal colour. ↑ urobilinogen.	Dark in colour.	Dark in colour. Absent urobilinogen.
Stool	Normal colour. ↑ urobilinogen.	Normal colour.	Pale colour. ↓ stercobilinogen.
ALP/GGT	↔	↑	↑↑
AST	↔	↑↑	↔/↑
PT	↔	↑ Not correctable with vitamin K.	↔ Correctable with vitamin K.

General surgery

> **1st line blood tests:**
> - **FBC:** Decreased haemoglobin if anaemia. May also see spherocyes or increased immature blood cells in the blood film in haemolytic anaemia.
> - **LFT:** See Table 5.2.
> - **Clotting screen:** Increased prothrombin time if hepatic or post-hepatic causes due to decreased synthesis of clotting factors.

Pre-hepatic cause suspected:
- **Blood film:** immature red cells (Reticulocytes), spherocytes or sickle cells may be seen.
- **Coombs test:** detects auto-antibodies to red blood cells.
- **Haptoglobin level:** bind to free haemoglobin and are therefore level is decreased in haemodialysis.

Hepatic cause suspected:
- **Viral titres:** HAV, HBV, HCV, CMV, EBV
- **Albumin level:** decreased due to decreased hepatic synthesis.
- **Prothrombin time:** prolonged due to reduced synthesis of clotting factors.
- **GGT level:** raised (more specific marker of hepatocyte damage than other transaminases).
- **Liver biopsy:** for tissue analysis if hepatitis suspected.
- **Ultrasound:** to visualise hepatic parenchyma.
- **CT/MRI:** to visualise intrahepatic masses.

Post-hepatic cause suspected:
- **ALP level:** raised as produced by cells lining the bile cannaliculi.
- **Ultrasound:** to visualise pathology.
- **CT:** to visualise pathology.
- **ERCP/MRCP:** to visualise pathology (can also stent bile duct with ERCP).

Figure 5.4 Investigation of jaundice.

5.5 GALLSTONES

5.5.1 EPIDEMIOLOGY

- Gallstones are common:
  - 10% of people over 50 years have gallstones.
  - Incidence increases with age.
- Affects more women than men 2F:1M.

5.5.2 AETIOLOGY

- Three types of gallstones:
  - Cholesterol stones (20%).
  - Bile pigment stones (5%).
  - Mixed stones (75%).
- See Figure 5.5.

5.5.3 CLINICAL FEATURES

- 80% are asymptomatic.
- There are several clinical presentations associated with gallstones (see Figure 5.6).

General surgery

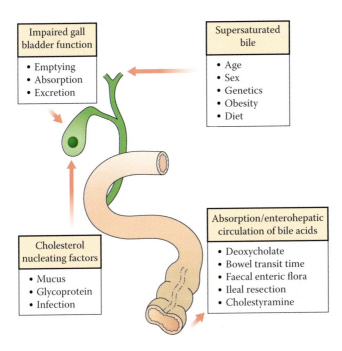

Figure 5.5 Factors associated with gallstone formation. (From: *Bailey & Love's Short Practice of Surgery, 26th Edition*, Figure 67.26, p. 1107.)

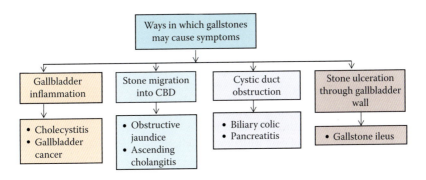

Figure 5.6 Causes of symptomatic gallstones.

Biliary colic

- Pain occurring when the gallbladder contracts against an obstruction (e.g. a stone in Hartmann's pouch or the cystic duct).
- Severe right upper quadrant (RUQ)/epigastric pain, lasting for a few hours.
- Usually precipitated by eating (often fatty foods).
- May be associated with nausea ± vomiting.
- Patient is usually systemically well (in contrast to acute cholecystitis).

General surgery

MICRO-print

Cholecystokinin is a hormone produced by the duodenum and small intestine in response to fat within the bowel lumen that causes gallbladder contraction.

Acute cholecystitis

- Prolonged gallbladder outlet obstruction, resulting in inflammation due to concentrated bile, initially resulting in chemical cholecystitis.
  - May subsequently be complicated by infection, pus (empyema) or mucus (mucocele).
- Often a history of previous biliary colic.
- RUQ/epigastric pain that becomes more severe, constant and localised after a day or two.
- Associated fever, ↑WCC, may be rigors and other features of sepsis.
- On examination there will be tenderness and guarding in the RUQ.
  - Murphy's sign positive.

MICRO-facts

Positive Murphy's sign: Ask the patient to take a deep breath in whilst placing your palpating hand below the costal margin in the RUQ. In acute gallbladder inflammation, the patient will "catch" his or her breath as the gallbladder descends during inspiration and comes into contact with the examining fingers, causing pain.

Chronic cholecystitis

- Repeated episodes of inflammation resulting in chronic fibrosis and thickening of the entire gallbladder wall.
- Recurrent episodes of pain with or without fever.

Acute obstructive jaundice

- Resulting from stones in the common bile duct (CBD): choledocholithiasis.
- Painful jaundice. (Painless jaundice is more usually due to malignant obstruction of the CBD: see Section 5.7.3).
- Usually acute onset and associated with pain.
- Can result in hepato-renal syndrome, resulting in acute renal failure.
- May cause a coagulopathy.

Gallstone pancreatitis

- CBD stones may cause acute pancreatitis (see Section 5.6).

Ascending cholangitis

- Infection of the bile in an obstructed ductal system.
- Occurs when biliary drainage is obstructed (usually by a CBD stone) and superadded infection occurs.
- Clinical symptoms are RUQ pain, fever and jaundice (Charcot's triad).
- ↑ WCC, features of sepsis, patients can become very sick very quickly.
- Monitor for renal failure and coagulopathy.
- Requires prompt diagnosis and treatment with early administration of antibiotics and urgent biliary drainage with either ERCP or a percutaneous stent.

Gallstone ileus

- Perforation of an inflamed gallbladder forming a cholecysto-enteric fistula, resulting in a large gallstone becoming lodged in the GI tract (usually in the distal small bowel as the calibre of the small bowel narrows progressively toward the ileocaecal valve).
- Features are of small bowel obstruction (may be a history of RUQ pain).
- Imaging may reveal a RIF opacity with air in the biliary tree (pneumobilia).
- Requires laparotomy, enterotomy and removal of the gallstone(s).
    - The gallbladder should not be removed. It has effectively treated itself by creating a wide-calibre drainage route for bile and gallstones and is usually part of an inflammatory mass making attempted surgical removal difficult and likely to cause more damage.

5.5.4 DIAGNOSIS

- Inflammatory markers (WCC, CRP) will usually be elevated in acute cholecystitis, cholangitis and pancreatitis.
- LFTs may show an obstructed picture. Serial measurements should be taken if obstructive jaundice is present to ensure its resolution or prompt further treatment if it remains elevated.
- Ultrasound scan (USS) is used to visualise the gallbladder and biliary tree, allowing diagnosis of stones, inflammation and duct dilatation.
- Plain abdominal x-ray is useful in gallstone ileus, as there will be evidence of small bowel obstruction, often with pneumobilia.
- MRCP allows better visualisation of the biliary tree and will demonstrate any gallstones within the CBD that may be causing obstruction (Figure 5.7), which will require removal (e.g. with ERCP or at surgery).
- ERCP is diagnostic for biliary tree dilatation and CBD stones, and is used therapeutically to remove obstructing CBD stones, insert stents and perform sphincterotomy (sphincter of Oddi).

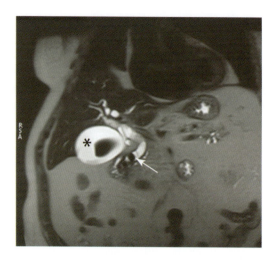

Figure 5.7 MRCP showing stone in the common bile duct (arrow) as well as a stone in the gallbladder (*). (From: *Browse's Introduction to the Investigation and Management of Surgical Disease*, Figure 18.19, p. 440.)

5.5.5 TREATMENT

Supportive measures

- Intravenous fluids and analgesia.
- Antibiotics are required in patients with acute cholecystitis, cholangitis and acute severe pancreatitis.
- Vitamin K is used to correct coagulopathy caused by obstructive jaundice.

ERCP may be used therapeutically in the presence of CBD obstruction

- Trawling of the duct to remove stones.
- Sphincterotomy to prevent further obstructive episodes.
- Insertion of stents to allow bile drainage in difficult cases.
- Complications include:
  - Bleeding, infection (cholangitis), pancreatitis, perforation.
- Percutaneous transhepatic cholangiography (PTC) is used in patients with severe biliary obstruction and sepsis who are unsuitable for ERCP or where it has been unsuccessful.
- Insertion of a percutaneous stent may relieve obstruction until sepsis subsides and the patient is well enough for alternative management.

Cholecystectomy

- Indications:
  - Acute or chronic cholecystitis, recurrent biliary colic, gallstone-induced pancreatitis, biliary peritonitis due to perforation of the gallbladder or previous CBD obstruction.

- Usually performed laparoscopically.
- Conversion to open procedure is rare and should occur in <5% of elective cases and <10% of emergency cases.
- May be a day-case procedure in simple elective cases.
- There is evidence to suggest that index admission laparoscopic cholecystectomy (i.e. on the patient's first admission with symptoms) is safe, prevents readmission and shortens overall hospital stay.
- On-table cholangiogram and duct exploration may be performed during laparoscopic cholecystectomy to identify and remove any stones.

MICRO-print

Other treatments for gallstones are rarely used but include:
- oral dissolution with chenodeoxycholic acid;
- lithotripsy.

MICRO-case

A 67-year-old female with known gallstones presents to the emergency department with RUQ pain and malaise. She is pyrexial, with signs of shock, and is obviously jaundiced. On questioning it is revealed she has recently noticed her urine is much darker and her stools paler.

This woman has presented with Charcot's triad of symptoms. She has ascending cholangitis.

Her blood results are shown below:

WCC	25.0×10^9/L	Amylase	51 iU/L
Bilirubin	302 mmol/L	GGT	562 g/L
ALP	825 iU/L	Creatinine	253 mmol/L
Urea	16.7 iU/L	INR	2.3

She has hepato-renal syndrome and requires IV fluid resuscitation. She also has deranged clotting as a result of the obstructive jaundice that requires correction with vitamin K. She is septic and should have immediate administration of IV antibiotics. Definitive management will include ERCP to remove the obstructing gallstone and allow drainage of the infected bile.

Learning points:
- Patients with ascending cholangitis can get very unwell very quickly and should be promptly diagnosed and managed.
- Patients with obstructive jaundice should have their clotting and renal function monitored regularly.
- Gallstones may present with a variety of clinical syndromes.

General surgery

5.6 ACUTE PANCREATITIS

5.6.1 PANCREATIC FUNCTION

- The pancreas has both exocrine and endocrine functions (Figure 5.8).

> **MICRO-print**
> Trypsinogen is converted to trypsin by enterokinase in the duodenum. Trypsin converts the inactive proenzymes into their active form.

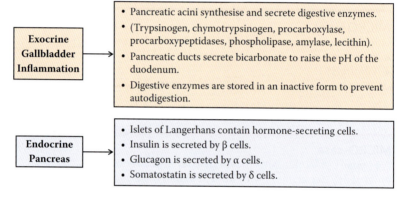

Figure 5.8 Pancreatic function.

5.6.2 DEFINITION

- Acute pancreatitis is an acute inflammation of the pancreas gland with an associated rise in serum pancreatic enzymes, which typically presents with severe abdominal pain. Chronic pancreatitis will be dealt with later in the chapter (see Section 5.6.10).

5.6.3 AETIOLOGY

- Peak incidence is at 60 years of age.
- Gallstone pancreatitis is more common in women, while alcohol-related pancreatitis is more common in men.
- Figure 5.9 shows the aetiological factors and their relative frequencies.

5.6.4 PATHOLOGY

- Acinar damage is caused by activation of pancreatic pro-enzymes, due to either:
  - hypersecretion with ductal obstruction or
  - reflux of duodenal contents into the pancreatic ducts.

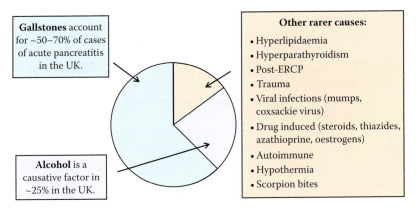

Gallstones account for ~50–70% of cases of acute pancreatitis in the UK.

Other rarer causes:
- Hyperlipidaemia
- Hyperparathyroidism
- Post-ERCP
- Trauma
- Viral infections (mumps, coxsackie virus)
- Drug induced (steroids, thiazides, azathioprine, oestrogens)
- Autoimmune
- Hypothermia
- Scorpion bites

Alcohol is a causative factor in ~25% in the UK.

Figure 5.9 Causes of pancreatitis and their frequencies.

- Auto-digestion ensues with further acinar damage, inflammation and injury to blood vessels, which may result in ischaemia and haemorrhage.
- Trypsin, lipase and amylase leak into the bloodstream, causing systemic effects.

5.6.5 CLINICAL FEATURES

Symptoms
- Acute onset epigastric pain that radiates to the back. Usually constant in nature and may be partially relieved by leaning forward.
- Nausea and vomiting.

Signs
- Abdominal examination will reveal a tender epigastrium and there may be local guarding or generalised rigidity.
- Abdominal distension with absent bowel sounds.
- There may be associated jaundice from biliary obstruction due to gallstones, local oedema or concurrent liver disease in alcoholic patients.
- Patients may demonstrate signs of shock due to dehydration (vomiting, anorexia), paralytic ileus (see Section 11.4) and fluid accumulation in the peritoneum and retroperitoneum and systemic inflammatory response syndrome (SIRS) (see Section 11.2) caused by release of vasoactive substances from the pancreas.
- Very rarely there may be signs of haemorrhagic pancreatitis due to the retroperitoneal spread of blood to these areas:
  - Grey Turner's sign: Bluish discolouration in the flank.
  - Cullen's sign: Bluish discolouration in the periumbilical area.

General surgery

Metabolic features

- Pancreatitis can result in severe metabolic disturbances so there may be clinical evidence of:
    - hypocalcaemia due to calcium sequestration in saponified fat in the abdomen secondary to the action of lipases;
    - hyperglycaemia due to damage to the pancreatic islet cells;
    - hypomagnesaemia.

5.6.6 DIAGNOSIS

- Serum amylase will be elevated to three to four times the upper limit of normal; over 1000 iU is diagnostic.
    - Serum amylase begins to fall 3–4 days after onset of pancreatitis and so patients presenting after 4–5 days of pain may not have a raised amylase.
        - As excretion of amylase is urinary, patients in this category may still have an elevated urinary amylase.
    - Patients with chronic inflammation may not demonstrate a rise in serum enzymes due to glandular destruction.
    - Serum lipase is less commonly used but has a longer half-life than amylase and has greater sensitivity and specificity.

Other blood tests

- CRP > 150 mg/dL is an independent indicator of severe acute pancreatitis.
- ↑ WCC due to inflammation ± secondary infection.
- Urea and electrolytes (U&E) may reveal dehydration or acute renal failure.
- LFTs may demonstrate an obstructive pattern.
- Blood glucose levels should be monitored.
- In addition, scoring systems are used to determine severity (see MICRO-FACTS box).

Imaging

- Erect chest x-ray (CXR) to rule out perforation as a cause of acute abdomen. It may also reveal lower lobe consolidation of the lung from local inflammation.
- Abdominal x-ray (AXR) may reveal evidence of paralytic ileus secondary to the severe peritoneal inflammation or occasionally a 'ground glass' appearance due to reactive ascites. A 'sentinel loop' of small bowel (focal duodenal ileus) may also be seen.
- USS identifies gallstones as a cause, assesses for CBD dilatation and the need for urgent ERCP.
- Contrast-enhanced computed tomography (CT) will demonstrate the pancreas more clearly, allowing assessment of the extent and whether there is necrosis of the pancreatic tissue that indicates a severe attack.

General surgery

> **MICRO-facts**
>
> Modified (Imrie) Glasgow criteria are used to assess the severity of acute pancreatitis. They are performed on admission, and again at 48 hours:
> - Age > 55 years.
> - WCC > 15×10^9/L.
> - Blood glucose > 10 mmol/L.
> - LDH > 600 iU/L.
> - Serum urea > 16 mmol/L.
> - PaO_2 < 8 kPa.
> - Calcium < 2 mmol/L.
> - Albumin < 32 g/L.
>
> Three or more positive criteria constitute a severe attack. These patients should undergo early CT scanning and be considered for admission to critical care.

5.6.7 TREATMENT

- Immediate resuscitation and assessment.
  - Analgesia.
  - IV fluids.
  - Oxygen.
  - Catheterisation and monitoring of urine output.
- The treatment of acute pancreatitis is mainly supportive. Patients may require the following additional treatments and regular assessment is needed to determine this.
  - Sliding scale insulin if blood glucose is elevated.
  - Nasogastric or total parenteral nutrition.
  - Antibiotics.
    - There is no evidence for the routine use of antibiotics in the treatment of pancreatitis, but many clinicians will give broad-spectrum cover for severe attacks and when there is evidence of necrosis or proven bacterial infection.
  - Replacement of electrolytes (e.g. magnesium, calcium).
  - Patients requiring intensive treatment unit (ITU) admission are likely to also require:
    - CVP monitoring and inotropes;
    - ventilatory support;
    - renal support via haemofiltration.
- ERCP may be indicated if there is an impacted bile duct stone.
- Surgery is very rarely needed and best avoided unless:
  - There is continued deterioration in the presence of severe necrotic pancreatitis.
  - Operable complications develop such as infected necrosis or chronic pseudocyst.

General surgery

MICRO-reference

British Society of Gastroenterology guidelines. UK guidelines for the management of acute pancreatitis. *GUT* 2005; 54: 1–9. http://www.bsg.org.uk/images/stories/docs/clinical/guidelines/pancreatic/pancreatic.pdf

MICRO-case

A 41-year-old female presents to her GP with intermittent RUQ pain that is precipitated by food and lasts up to an hour. FBC and LFTs are normal. An USS reveals gallstones. She is referred for cholecystectomy.

She subsequently attends the emergency department with severe epigastric pain, radiating to her back, and vomiting. She is pyrexial, slightly hypotensive and appears mildly jaundiced. Her blood results are shown below:

WCC	18.0×10^9/L	Amylase	1021 iU/L
CRP	200 mg/dL	LDH	652 iU/L
Bilirubin	175 mmol/L	Albumin	41 g/L
ALP	634 iU/L	Calcium	2.1 mmol/L
GGT	451 iU/L	Urea	9.5 mmol/L
Glucose	6.5 mmol/L	PaO_2	7.9 kPa

She has acute severe gallstone pancreatitis (she scores 3 on the modified Glasgow score). She is managed on the HDU with IV fluid resuscitation, IV antibiotics, NBM, strict fluid balance and vitamin K. USS shows a gallstone within a newly dilated CBD. She undergoes urgent ERCP to relieve the obstruction and her condition improves.

Learning points:

- Pancreatitis is a potentially life-threatening condition, even in young patients, and should be treated as such.
- Gallstones may present with a variety of clinical syndromes.

5.6.8 COMPLICATIONS

Infected pancreatic necrosis

- Bacterial infection of a severely inflamed and necrotic pancreas usually leads to generalised sepsis and multi-organ failure and may require surgical necrosectomy.

Haemorrhagic pancreatitis

- Erosion of local blood vessels can result in haemorrhage and is associated with Cullen's and Grey Turner's signs. This usually denotes a more severe attack with a higher mortality.

General surgery

Pseudoaneurysm

- Damage to local blood vessels may result in pseudoaneurysm formation that can subsequently bleed, resulting in often life-threatening haemorrhage.
- Early detection and radiological embolisation are essential to prevent death.

Pseudocyst

- Persistent collection of amylase-rich fluid, enclosed in a wall of fibrous or granulation tissue.
- May cause persistent epigastric pain and a palpable epigastric mass.
- Most resolve spontaneously over time, but persistent or symptomatic cysts may require percutaneous, endoscopic or operative drainage.

Systemic complications

- Organ dysfunction may occur and is life-threatening, requiring HDU/ICU support:
  - Respiratory, cardiac, renal, malnutrition, systemic inflammatory response syndrome, coagulopathy/disseminated intravascular coagulation (DIC), multi-organ failure.
- Chronic diabetes mellitus and pancreatic exocrine insufficiency may rarely follow a particularly severe attack.

5.6.9 PROGNOSIS

- Overall mortality of acute pancreatitis is ~5%.
- The presence of organ failure increases mortality.
- With acute haemorrhagic pancreatitis mortality is in excess of 30%.

5.6.10 CHRONIC PANCREATITIS

- Chronic pancreatitis is a continuing inflammatory process that results in continuing pain, permanent loss of function and is characterised by irreversible damage to the gland.
- It is more common with alcohol-related pancreatitis where there have been recurrent attacks.
- There is damage to the acini and destruction of the gland parenchyma with subsequent fibrosis and ductal stenosis.
- Clinically the presentation is with pain, nausea and vomiting, similar to that of acute pancreatitis. There may also be:
  - Weight loss.
  - Steatorrhoea.
  - Insulin-dependent diabetes occurs in 30–40%.
- Imaging of the pancreas often reveals calcification of the gland.
- Treatment in the acute phase is largely conservative.
- In the long term, treatment consists of:
  - total abstinence from alcohol;
  - low-fat diet;

General surgery

- pancreatic enzyme replacement (e.g. Creon™);
- insulin therapy for diabetes mellitus;
- administration of fat-soluble vitamins.
- Pain control is often difficult in these patients, with many becoming narcotic dependent. Chronic pain teams are useful and difficult cases should be managed in a specialised unit.

5.7 PANCREATIC MALIGNANCIES

5.7.1 EPIDEMIOLOGY

- Pancreatic carcinoma is the 10th most common cancer in the UK but the 5th leading cause of cancer death due to its persisting high percentage mortality.

5.7.2 PATHOLOGY

- Adenocarcinoma is the most common histological type (96%).
- Categorised by site: Head of the pancreas (65%), body (25%), tail (10%).

5.7.3 CLINICAL FEATURES

Carcinoma of the head of the pancreas

- Obstructive jaundice.
- It is often painless but pain is sometimes present, usually epigastric or left upper quadrant and may radiate to the back.
  - It is described as 'deep' or 'gnawing' and is constant.
  - In contrast, the pain of acute gallstone-induced obstructive jaundice is severe and of sudden onset.
- An abdominal mass may be palpable due to the tumour itself; hepatomegaly due to metastasis or the gallbladder may be palpable.
- Other non-specific symptoms include anorexia, nausea, vomiting, weight loss (present in 80% of cases), fatigue, malaise, pruritis.
- Acute pancreatitis may sometimes be the presenting feature.
- Thrombophlebitis migrans (10% of cases)—venous thrombosis associated with a hypercoagulable state. May also present with embolic events.

MICRO-facts

Courvoisier's law: A palpable gallbladder in the presence of jaundice is unlikely to be due to gallstones.
- In stone disease, the gallbladder is usually diseased and so doesn't greatly distend. However, with other causes of obstructive jaundice (e.g. carcinoma of the head of the pancreas), the normal gallbladder is able to distend and so is felt as a palpable RUQ mass.

Carcinoma of the body and tail

- More likely to be asymptomatic until the disease is more advanced.
- Epigastric pain relieved on leaning forward is a common feature.
- Significant weight loss.
- A palpable epigastric mass.
- Obstructive jaundice occurs late, due to metastasis or lymph node spread.
- Thrombophlebitis migrans.
- Diabetes mellitus.

Signs

- Jaundice.
- Weight loss.
- Abdominal mass.
- Virchow's node (left-sided supraclavicular lymph node) may be present.

5.7.4 DIAGNOSIS

- Blood tests: full blood count (FBC), LFT, blood sugar, inflammatory markers (e.g. ESR).
- Tumour markers. CA19-9 has a high sensitivity for pancreatic carcinoma, but has a high false positive rate. It can also be used in treatment monitoring.

Imaging

- USS initially, but it is less sensitive in body and tail tumours.
- CT or endoscopic US scanning is used to demonstrate the tumour, and assess disease spread, e.g. liver metastasis and invasion of the superior mesenteric vessels.
- MRCP may give better visualisation of the anatomy and operability, especially relating to invasion of the mesenteric vessels.
- Biopsy should not be performed, unless endoscopic, if surgery is being considered.

5.7.5 TREATMENT

- Only around 15–20% of patients present with resectable disease, but this is often complicated by the patient being unfit for major surgery.
- All patients require MDT input.
- Where resection is possible a pancreatico-duodenectomy (either a pylorus-preserving pancreatico-duodenectomy (PPPD) or the more traditional Whipple's procedure) is the best option for pancreatic head and neck cancers, but carries a high operative morbidity and mortality (approaching 5%) with a 5-year survival of only 15–20%.
    - This is a complicated procedure involving proximal partial pancreatectomy, with distal choledochectomy and cholecystectomy, and a Roux-en-Y anastomosis plus or minus a distal gastrectomy.

- For the rarely operable cancers of the body and tail, distal pancreatectomy with en bloc splenectomy is appropriate.
- Further management:
  - Post-operative chemotherapy provides an increased survival benefit using fluorouracil (5FU) and folinic acid (or trials of gemcitabine/capecitabine).
- For those with inoperable disease:
  - Palliative ERCP with stenting of the compressed bile duct.
  - Percutaneous transhepatic cholangiogram (PTC) with stenting may also be used.
  - Occasionally surgical bypass may be required.
  - Palliative care input is often needed to control abdominal pain.
  - Pancreatic failure also needs management for both pancreatic endocrine and exocrine functions.
  - There is also a role for palliative chemotherapy with gemcitabine.

5.7.6 PROGNOSIS

- The 5-year survival of pancreatic carcinoma is around 2%, and currently the only available option to improve survival is surgical (5-year survival for resectable disease is still only 12%).
  - The majority of patients receive palliative therapy, and the average survival from diagnosis still remains approximately 6 months.

MICRO-print

Neuroendocrine tumours of the pancreas can occur, with an incidence of 1 in 100 000. These most commonly present with symptoms of ectopic hormone secretion. The types of tumour seen are insulinoma, gastrinoma (Zollinger-Ellison syndrome), VIPoma, glucagonoma and somatostatinoma.

5.8 PRIMARY HEPATIC MALIGNANCIES

- Known as hepatocellular carcinoma (HCC).

5.8.1 AETIOLOGY

- The main causal factors are those of an established liver pathology, and 80% of HCC are found in patients with cirrhosis, which may be due to:
  - hepatitis B and C viruses;
  - alcoholic cirrhosis;
  - haemochromatosis;
  - chronic hepatitis.

> **MICRO-facts**
>
> HCC occurs in 25% of patients with alcoholic cirrhosis for over 5 years.

- Males are more commonly affected.
- Other diseases associated with HCC are:
  - primary sclerosing cholangitis;
  - α1-antitrypsin deficiency;
  - porphyria cutanea tarda.
- There is also an association with androgenic steroids and oral contraceptive use.

5.8.2 EPIDEMIOLOGY

- The incidence of HCC demonstrates marked geographic variation due to its aetiological factors.
  - It is most common in Asia and Africa, but rare in the UK.

5.8.3 CLINICAL FEATURES

- This varies depending on whether or not liver disease is already present.
  - In the absence of cirrhosis it may present with hepatomegaly and ascites.
  - In the presence of liver disease, presentation is with rapid deterioration of symptoms with anorexia, weight loss, fever and right upper quadrant pain.
- There may be stigmata of cirrhosis, and a tender, enlarged and irregular liver edge.

5.8.4 DIAGNOSIS

- Serum α-fetoprotein (AFP) may be raised, but is normal in a third of patients, and cirrhosis itself is associated with an increase in AFP also.
- USS of the liver may show the tumour or a change in the size or positioning of the liver, and may demonstrate filling defects. It will also aid guidance for biopsy.
- CT scanning will identify any liver masses. Like ultrasound, any lesion smaller than 1 cm cannot reliably be differentiated from nodular cirrhosis.
- Magnetic resonance imaging (MRI) scanning is the main imaging modality for determination of operability.
- Liver biopsy should never be performed prior to MDT review of the case to determine whether surgery is possible, due to the risk of seeding along the needle tract.

5.8.5 TREATMENT

- This is dependent on the number and size of tumours present, the patient's co-morbidities, and the presence or absence of cirrhosis and metastases.
  - If the lesion(s) is small and localised, curative resection can be attempted.
  - If the tumour meets the Milan criteria (tumours less than 5 cm and fewer than 3 present), then transplantation may have a good outcome.
- Chemo-embolisation or radiofrequency ablation may be used in selected patients.

5.8.6 PROGNOSIS

- As HCC often presents late, the prognosis is poor, often only about 6 months.

MICRO-print

Fibrolamellar carcinoma: This does not present on the background of liver disease. It is commoner in younger patients (young adults and children), and is seen as a large vascular mass.

5.9 SECONDARY HEPATIC MALIGNANCIES

5.9.1 PATHOLOGY

- The most common primary sites metastasising to the liver are the GI tract (e.g. stomach and colon), the breast and bronchus.
  - GI liver metastases are thought to occur via the portal venous system.

5.9.2 CLINICAL FEATURES

- Clinical features may be divided into those of the primary tumour, systemic features and those from the liver itself (Figure 5.10).

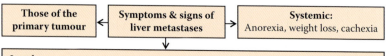

Those of the primary tumour	→	Symptoms & signs of liver metastases	→	Systemic: Anorexia, weight loss, cachexia

Local:
Hepatomegaly with a hard, irregular edge. Abdominal pain. Hepatic failure. Jaundice occurs late due to destruction of the liver tissue and bile duct compression. Portal vein compression causes varices and ascites. IVC compression causes leg oedema.

Figure 5.10 Clinical features of liver metastases.

5.9.3 DIAGNOSIS

- LFTs may show ↑ALP, ↑bilirubin, ↓albumin.
- Carcinoembryonic antigen (CEA) is ↑ in 75% of patients with colonic metastases.
- Imaging of the liver with either ultrasound or CT scanning (Figure 5.11).
- MRI is the gold standard for assessing operability.
- Biopsy is contra-indicated prior to MDT discussion to prevent the risk of seeding of the needle track.
- Identification of the primary with either CT of the chest abdomen and pelvis, breast examination in females and in some cases a positron emission tomography (PET) scan.

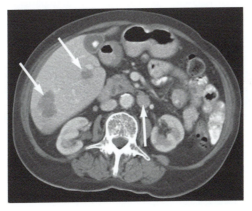

Figure 5.11 Axial CT showing secondary deposits in the liver (two arrows) and enlarged para-aortic lymph nodes (single arrow). (From: *Illustrated Clinical Anatomy, 2nd Edition*, Figure 7.7, p. 103.)

5.9.4 TREATMENT

- This is dependent on the extent of metastases, condition of the patient and the type and operability of the primary tumour.
- 10–20% of patients with liver metastases from colonic origin may be suitable for metastasectomy with curative intent.
  - Metastatic disease of breast, gastric, pancreatic or lung origin is not suitable for surgical resection.
- Pre-operative chemotherapy may be used to downsize the tumour and enhance operability.
- Up to 70% of the liver may be resected if no other liver disease is present.
  - Resection is usually considered in young patients with up to four lesions within one lobe.
- Renal cell carcinoma and neuroendocrine tumour liver metastases may also be resectable. For most other primary tumours liver metastases represent surgically incurable disease.

General surgery

- For patients with inoperable liver metastases from colorectal cancer, palliative chemotherapy may confer significant improvements in survival.
  - Regimes including various combinations of capecitabine, irinotecan, oxaliplatin and cetuximab may all be used.
  - For other primary sites, other chemotherapy regimes may be helpful.
- Dexamethasone may help with liver capsular pain.
- Palliative care involvement for pain control, pruritis, as well as nutritional, social and emotional support is vital.

5.9.5 PROGNOSIS

- Life expectancy for most patients is less than 2 years.
  - However there is a 35–40% 5-year survival in patients with resectable metastatic colon cancer.

> **MICRO-facts**
>
> More than 25% of patients who die of malignant disease have hepatic secondaries. More than 90% of patients with hepatic metastasis have metastatic disease elsewhere.

5.10 BILIARY MALIGNANCIES: GALLBLADDER

5.10.1 AETIOLOGY

- 70–85% are associated with gallstones.
  - This may be due to irritation of the gallbladder or a carcinogenic effect of components of the stones.
- Cancers are found in 50% of 'porcelain gallbladders' (chronic cholecystitis with diffuse calcification) on histology following cholecystectomy.
- Polyps of the gallbladder may also be pre-cancerous.
- It is associated with ulcerative colitis and primary sclerosing cholangitis.

> **MICRO-print**
>
> Benign gallbladder polyps are common. They may be inflammatory or composed of cholesterol. Cholecystectomy is recommended for any polyp of >1 cm in diameter due to the risk of malignant transformation.

5.10.2 EPIDEMIOLOGY

- Constitute about 1% of all cancers.
- Occurs most commonly in patients aged 60–70.
- Affects women three times more commonly than men.

General surgery

5.10.3 PATHOLOGY

- 90% are adenocarcinomas, with 10% being squamous cell carcinomas.
- There is often direct spread to the liver.
- There may also be lymphatic spread to the hilar lymph nodes or haematogenous spread to distant sites.

5.10.4 CLINICAL FEATURES

- Presentation is similar to chronic cholecystitis, with right upper quadrant pain, nausea and vomiting.
- There may be significant weight loss and obstructive jaundice in the later stages.
- Gallbladder cancer is often found incidentally at the time of elective cholecystectomy, and this may be curative if performed prior to local spread.

5.10.5 DIAGNOSIS

- USS or CT scan may reveal a gallbladder mass and demonstrate disease extent.
- CA19-9 and CEA may be raised.
- ERCP may be performed if the patient requires a stent to allow the flow of bile.

5.10.6 TREATMENT

- If disease is confined to the gallbladder, then cholecystectomy is curative; however this is rarely the case.
- Wide local excision may be performed if there is direct spread to the liver.
- If there is lymphatic or biliary tree involvement, curative surgery is not possible.
- A small minority are sensitive to radiotherapy, but they are not chemosensitive.

5.10.7 PROGNOSIS

- Poor with a less than 5% 5-year survival rate.

5.11 BILIARY MALIGNANCIES: CHOLANGIOCARCINOMA

5.11.1 AETIOLOGY

- Cholangiocarcinomas are rare tumours of the biliary tree and are associated with:
  - Primary sclerosing cholangitis and inflammatory bowel disease.
  - Congenital hepatic abnormalities.
  - Chronic biliary infection.

General surgery

5.11.2 PATHOLOGY

- They are composed of mucin-secreting cells and are adenocarcinomas.
- Spread is usually lymphatic or by local extension.

5.11.3 CLINICAL FEATURES

- Painless obstructive jaundice.
- Other symptoms include weight loss, steatorrhoea and epigastric pain.
- On examination, there may be hepatomegaly but no palpable gallbladder, as the obstruction is proximal.

5.11.4 DIAGNOSIS

- Imaging with USS, CT or MRCP may demonstrate changes in the biliary tree.
- Biopsy confirmation by CT-guided PTC or ERCP.
  - Percutaneous biopsy should only be performed following MDT discussion due to the risk of seeding cancer cells along the biopsy needle tract.

5.11.5 TREATMENT

- Localised disease is treated surgically, with partial hepatic resection.
- Palliative relief of bile duct obstruction, usually with stenting of the malignant stricture, improves quality of life and pain.

5.11.6 PROGNOSIS

- Although slow-growing and metastasising late, patients do not usually survive longer than 6 months from diagnosis.

6 Upper GI

6.1 GASTRO-OESOPHAGEAL REFLUX DISEASE (GORD)

- The surface anatomy of the gastrointestinal tract is shown in Figure 6.1.

6.1.1 DEFINITION

- Reflux of gastric contents into the oesophagus causing irritation and inflammation.

6.1.2 EPIDEMIOLOGY

- Common—occurs in up to 5% of normal individuals.
- More common in middle age.

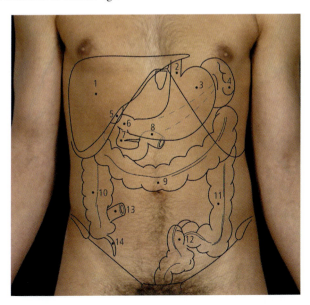

Figure 6.1 Surface anatomy of the GI tract. (From: *Illustrated Clinical Anatomy, 2nd Edition*, Figure 5.2, p. 76.)

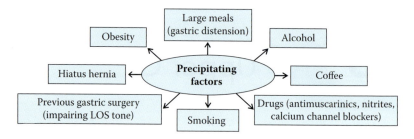

Figure 6.2 Precipitants of GORD.

6.1.3 AETIOLOGY

- Complex mix of:
  - Hypotonia of the lower oesophageal sphincter (LOS).
  - Reduced oesophageal peristalsis (with decreased acid clearance).
  - Impairment of the pinch-cock effect of the diaphragm on the lower oesophagus.
  - Delayed gastric emptying with increased intragastric pressure.
- Precipitating factors are shown in Figure 6.2.

6.1.4 CLINICAL FEATURES

Dyspepsia

- Usually retrosternal and can radiate to the neck, left arm and epigastrium.
  - Important as can be mistaken for cardiac pain.
- Worse on bending, lying, after a large meal, on consumption of alcohol or hot liquids.

Regurgitation

- Worse on bending and lying.
- May be just acid or gastric contents (i.e. food).

6.1.5 DIAGNOSIS

- OGD to assess severity of oesophagitis (with biopsies if indicated).
- Barium swallow and meal to look for hiatus hernia.

pH monitoring

- 24-hour monitoring with a probe in the oesophagus to assess the quantity and frequency of acid reflux (pH < 4).
- Can correlate the reflux episodes with symptoms.
- Indicated if surgical management is being considered.

General surgery

Oesophageal manometry

- To assess the motility of the oesophagus and LOS pressure.

6.1.6 MANAGEMENT

Pharmacotherapy

- Proton pump inhibitors (PPIs) (e.g. lansoprazole, omeprazole) are highly successful in the majority of patients.
- H2-antagonist may be used as second line (e.g. ranitidine).
- Alginate antacids (e.g. Gaviscon®) can provide symptomatic relief.
- Prokinetic dopamine antagonists (e.g. domperidone, metoclopramide) help by promoting gastric emptying and increasing the tone of the LOS.

Surgery

- Indicated if there is failure to respond to full-dose medical therapy, risk of aspiration pneumonia or severe complications are present.
- Laparoscopic Nissen's fundoplication:
  - Wrapping of the gastric fundus around the distal section of the oesophagus to increase the tone of the LOS.

MICRO-facts

General measures for management of GORD:
- Lose weight (especially if a hiatus hernia is present).
- Reduce alcohol and caffeine intake and stop smoking.
- Avoid eating meals within 3 hours of going to bed.
- Prop the head end of the bed up.

6.1.7 COMPLICATIONS

- Peptic stricture (see Figure 6.3):
  - More common in patients > 60 years.
  - Occurs on long background history of dysphagia.

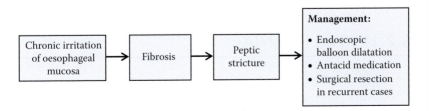

Figure 6.3 Aetiology and management of peptic strictures.

General surgery

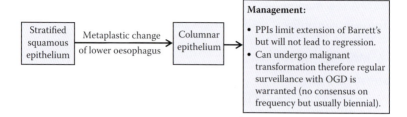

Figure 6.4 Aetiology and management of Barrett's oesophagus.

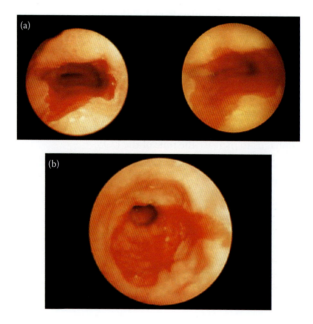

Figure 6.5 Barrett's oesophagus with proximal migration of the squamocolumnar junction. (From: *Bailey & Love's Short Practice of Surgery, 26th Edition*, Figure, 59.27, p. 1022.)

- Barrett's oesophagus (see Figures 6.4 and 6.5):
  - Affects ≤20% of patients with GORD.
  - More common in middle-aged male sufferers.

6.2 HIATUS HERNIA

6.2.1 DEFINITION

- Abnormal protrusion of the proximal part of the stomach through the diaphragmatic hiatus into the thorax.

6.2.2 EPIDEMIOLOGY

- Common; incidence increases with age.
- M:F = M < F.

6.2.3 CLINICAL FEATURES

- There are two main types of hiatus hernia (see Figure 6.6 and Table 6.1).

6.2.4 DIAGNOSIS

- Barium swallow to identify the type of hernia and assess the severity.

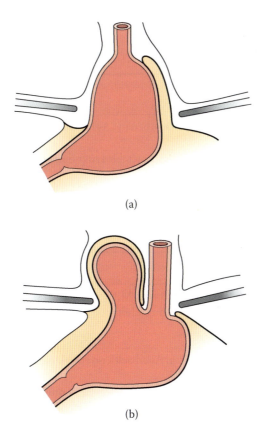

(a)

(b)

Figure 6.6 (a) Sliding and (b) rolling hiatus hernias. (From: *Browse's Introduction to the Investigation and Management of Surgical Disease*, Figure 18.11, p. 431.)

Table 6.1 Features of the different types of hiatus hernia.

CHARACTERISTIC	SLIDING	ROLLING
Epidemiology	~90% of herniae.	~10% of herniae.
Aetiology	Herniation of the gastro-oesophageal junction (GOJ) into the hernia, thus increasing the size of the hiatus.	Gastric herniation occurs but the GOJ remains below the diaphragm so part of the stomach lies alongside the distal part of the oesophagus.
Clinical features	Dyspepsia. Regurgitation.	Dyspepsia. Odynophagia (due to pressure from contents of hernia). 'Pressure in the chest'. Dyspnoea on eating and bending if severe (due to pressure from contents of hernia).

6.2.5 MANAGEMENT

- General measures and pharmacotherapy: As for GORD (see Section 6.1).
- Surgery:
  - Rarely performed unless intractable symptoms or volvulus in rolling type.
  - Laparoscopic fixation of stomach with plication of the diaphragm.
  - Nissen's fundoplication.

6.3 ACHALASIA

6.3.1 EPIDEMIOLOGY

- Prevalence = 0.5–1 per 100 000 with M:F = 2:3.
- Two peaks in age of onset—young adulthood and elderly.

6.3.2 AETIOLOGY

- Due to loss of ganglion cells in Auerbach's myenteric plexus causing failure of relaxation of the LOS.
- Results in progressive dilatation of the oesophagus proximal to the LOS.

6.3.3 CLINICAL FEATURES

- Dysphagia worse for liquids, then progressing to solids.
- Odynophagia (painful swallowing) in the early stage of the disease.
- Weight loss and anorexia.

General surgery

- Effortless regurgitation, especially on lying flat.
- Recurrent chest infections due to aspiration pneumonia.

6.3.4 DIAGNOSIS

OGD

- Will show a tight LOS with proximal dilation and pooling of food and fluid in the oesophagus.

CXR

- Widening of the mediastinum with a fluid level behind the heart.

Barium swallow and meal

- Failure of LOS relaxation with tapering of the distal oesophagus (appearance of a 'rat's tail'/'bird's beak' at LOS; see Figure 6.7).

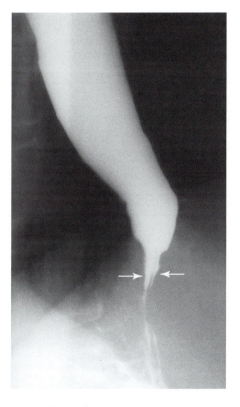

Figure 6.7 Barium swallow demonstrating a dilated oesophagus with the characteristic smooth stricture (bird's beak) of achalasia at its lower end. (From: *Browse's Introduction to the Investigation and Management of Surgical Disease*, Figure 18.3, p. 425.)

Oesophageal manometry

- Failure of LOS relaxation, decreased peristaltic activity and increased oesophageal pressure on swallowing.

6.3.5 MANAGEMENT

Pneumatic dilatation

- Endoscopically guided balloon dilatation.
- Commonly results in reflux symptoms and can rarely lead to perforation.

Heller's myotomy

- Surgical relief of increased tone by incising the LOS down to the mucosa.
- Highly successful, especially in young patients.
- Can lead to reflux symptoms post-surgery.

Botulinum injection

- Endoscopically guided injection into LOS causing interruption of the cholinergic activity and therefore decreased tone.
- Effects are not permanent, and therefore it needs to be repeated.

MICRO-facts

Achalasia can be associated with a malignant transformation (squamous cell carcinoma) in 2–7% of patients, and therefore periodical monitoring via OGD is necessary.

6.4 MALLORY–WEISS TEAR

6.4.1 DEFINITION

- Oesophageal trauma leading to a tear in the mucosal surface.

6.4.2 AETIOLOGY

- Caused by prolonged forceful vomiting.

6.4.3 CLINICAL FEATURES

- History of repeated forceful vomiting/retching.
- Haematemesis:
  - Streaks of red blood or 'coffee grounds' (dark brown flecks) in the vomit.

6.4.4 DIAGNOSIS

- OGD to rule out other causes of haemetemesis.

6.4.5 MANAGEMENT

- Usually resolves spontaneously within 14 days.
- Conservative use of antacids.
- May need fluid resuscitation and correction of electrolytes if hypotensive and there is a prolonged sickness precipitating the tear.

6.5 OESOPHAGEAL VARICES

6.5.1 DEFINITION

- Dilated oesophageal veins secondary to portal hypertension (i.e. portal pressure > 10–20 mmHg).
- Responsible for 20% of upper gastrointestinal (GI) bleeding.

6.5.2 AETIOLOGY

- Anything that causes portal hypertension:
  - hepatic cirrhosis (90% of sufferers will develop varices over 10 years);
  - portal vein obstruction, e.g. thrombosis, compression from tumour;
  - acute hepatitis;
  - schistosomiasis;
  - Budd–Chiari syndrome.

6.5.3 CLINICAL FEATURES

- Haematemesis:
  - Rupture of varices leads to acute (and often torrential) bleeding.
  - 1/3 of patients with varices will bleed.
- Abdominal pain.
- Dysphagia (uncommon).
- Clinical signs of haemorrhage, chronic liver disease or acute hepatic failure may be present (Figure 6.8).

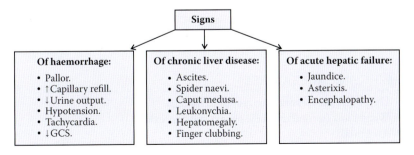

Figure 6.8 Signs that may be present in a patient with oesophageal varices.

General surgery

6.5.4 DIAGNOSIS

- Full blood count (FBC) may reveal a macrocytic anaemia secondary to alcoholism with platelets.
- Clotting screen and liver function tests (LFTs) may both be deranged secondary to liver disease.
- Urea and electrolytes (U&E) should be performed to assess dehydration.
- OGD will confirm the presence of the varices and assess severity.

6.5.5 MANAGEMENT

- Resuscitation and stabilisation (see Section 6.7).
- Endoscopic band ligation:
  - Occlusion of the varices by use of a band causing thrombosis.
  - Often needs to be repeated.
- Endoscopic sclerotherapy:
  - Injection of a sclerosing agent (e.g. ethanolamine oleate) into varices to promote thrombosis.
  - Successful in <80% of patients but may need repeating.
- Transjugular intrahepatic portosystemic shunt (TIPS):
  - Endovascular technique via the jugular vein.
  - Creates an artificial channel within the liver between the inflow portal vein and the outflow hepatic vein.
  - Decreases portal venous pressure, thereby lessening the pressure on the blood vessels (varices) so that bleeding is less likely to occur.
- Balloon tamponade is used for severe variceal bleeding if control cannot be gained with vasoconstrictor or endoscopic therapies.

6.6 OESOPHAGEAL CANCER

6.6.1 EPIDEMIOLOGY

- Ninth commonest cancer in the UK (accounts for 3% of cancers) (Figure 6.9).
- Incidence increases with age.

6.6.2 PATHOLOGY

- There are two pathological types of oesophageal cancer (see Table 6.2).

6.6.3 CLINICAL FEATURES

- Dysphagia progressing from solids to liquids.
- Weight loss (secondary to dysphagia and anorexia).
- Anaemia.
- Cervical lymphadenopathy (metastasis to nodes, e.g. Virchow's node).
- Hoarse voice and bovine cough (from invasion of the recurrent laryngeal nerve).

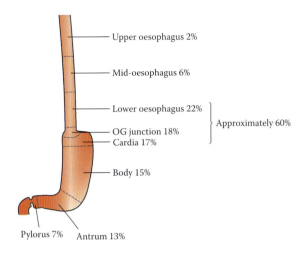

Upper oesophagus 2%

Mid-oesophagus 6%

Lower oesophagus 22%

OG junction 18%
Cardia 17%

Approximately 60%

Body 15%

Pylorus 7%   Antrum 13%

Figure 6.9 The distribution of upper gastrointestinal tract cancer in the UK. (From: *Bailey & Love's Short Practice of Surgery, 26th Edition*, Figure 60.25, p. 1068.)

Table 6.2 Epidemiology, aetiology and pathology of oesophageal cancer.

	SQUAMOUS CELL CARCINOMA	ADENOCARCINOMA
Epidemiology	M:F = 2:1. High incidence in China and parts of Africa.	M:F = 5:1. Incidence increasing in Western society.
Location	Generally occurs in the upper 2/3, although rare in the top 1/3.	Occurs in the lower 1/3.
Risk factors	Smoking. Alcohol. Diet, e.g. lack of vitamins and iron. Achalasia. Coeliac disease. Plummer-Vinson syndrome.	Smoking. Alcohol. Obesity. High dietary intake of nitrosamines. Long history of GORD. Barrett's oesophagus.

6.6.4 DIAGNOSIS

OGD
- May see a malignant stricture.
- Will need to take a biopsy to confirm diagnosis and grade.

Barium swallow
- May demonstrate an irregular narrowing.

General surgery

MICRO-print

Staging investigations for oesophageal cancer:

- **CT:** First-line investigation.
- **Endoluminal ultrasound:** To assess the depth of the tumour, local spread to lymph nodes and to perform a fine-needle aspiration.
- **Laparoscopic staging:** Performed prior to therapeutic surgery (if being considered) to assess for peritoneal or visceral metastases.

MICRO-facts

Staging and prognosis:

- Non-specific symptoms mean that patients with oesophageal cancer present at an advanced stage (70% present with stage 3 disease).
- Staging is done using the TNM system:

  T_{is} = carcinoma in situ.
  T_1 = invasion of lamina propria.
  T_2 = invasion of muscularis propria.
  T_3 = invasion of adventitia.
  T_4 = invasion of adjacent structures.

  N_0 = no nodes involved.
  N_1 = regional nodes involved.
  M_0 = no distant metastases.
  M_1 = distant metastases.

- 5-year survival:
  - Stage 1 (T_1, N_0, M_0) = 80%.
  - Stage 2 (T_{2-3}, N_0, M_0 or T_{1-2}, N_1, M_0) = 30%.
  - Stage 3 (T_3, N_1, M_0 or T_4, any N, M_0) = 18%.
  - Stage 4 (any T, any N, M_1) = 4%.

6.6.5 MANAGEMENT

Curative intent

- Ivor-Lewis procedure—laparotomy plus transthoracic oesophagectomy.
- Neoadjuvant or adjuvant chemotherapy (platinum based) may be useful.

Palliation

- Maintenance of luminal patency via endoscopic stenting.
- Endoscopic laser therapy can be used to ablate lesion to restore patency.
- External beam or intraluminal radiotherapy is used to relieve symptoms.

General surgery

6.7 HOW TO MANAGE ACUTE UPPER GI HAEMORRHAGE

6.7.1 PRESENTATION

- Haemetemesis (blood in the vomit).
- Melaena (altered blood in the stool, usually black and tarry).
- Fresh PR bleeding—rapid transit of an upper GI bleed may present as fresh blood per rectum.
- Shock.

> **MICRO-facts**
>
> The commonest cause of GI bleeding is peptic ulceration (~70%).

6.7.2 MANAGEMENT

- Take an ABCDE approach to managing patients with haematemesis.
  - Call for support early, e.g. from senior surgical and anaesthetic doctors.
  - Administer oxygen therapy.
  - Ensure adequate IV access (two large-bore cannulas).
    - At the same time draw off blood for FBC, U&E, LFTs, clotting and group and save or cross-match.
  - Preferably continuous monitoring or regular observations.
    - Monitor heart rate, blood pressure and capillary refill time.
    - Consider a catheter to monitor urine output.
  - Administer intravenous fluids.
    - Consider a fluid bolus if the patient is hypotensive or tachycardic.
    - Remember the patient may require a blood transfusion at this point—ensure it is available.
  - Administer an intravenous PPI.
  - Check the Hb level—if less than 8, request 2 units of whole blood.
    - In massive haemorrhage—request 6–8 units of whole blood.
    - Remember to repeat the Hb; a rapid drop indicates ongoing haemorrhage.

> **MICRO-print**
>
> If whole blood is unavailable, transfusion of packed red cells only in massive transfusion is inadequate. Platelets, Cryoprecipitate and Fresh Frozen Plasma (FFP) should also be administered to replace the losses of other blood components. Blood banks may supply, "massive transfusion packs" in these situations, providing all the components to be equivalent to a large transfusion of whole blood.

- Take a history, noting any clues to the source of bleeding:
  - Previous UGI bleed?

- Previous OGD—history of varices or ulcers?
- Medications—current non-steroidal anti-inflammatory drugs (NSAIDs), aspirin, warfarin, etc.
- Alcohol history, liver disease?
- Perform a thorough examination noting:
  - Signs of significant blood loss.
    - Pallor, capillary refill time, skin turgor.
  - Evidence of a bleeding tendency.
    - Purpura, bruising.
  - Pre-existing liver disease.
    - Jaundice, hepatomegaly, splenomegaly, spider naevi.
  - Remember to perform a PR to confirm the presence or absence of melaena.
- Further management may need instigating if the patient continues to actively bleed.
  - Upper GI endoscopy.
    - Allows visualisation of any lesions and often therapeutic interventions can be performed at the same time.
    - If a bleeding ulcer is seen, then this should be treated with injected adrenaline and vessel coagulation with heated probe or laser therapy.
    - If varices are the cause, these should be treated with injection sclerotherapy (to produce vessel thrombosis) or variceal banding.
  - The patient may require vasoconstrictor therapy to reduce splanchnic blood flow (with either terlipressin or somatostatin; evidence suggests mortality is not altered by these drugs).
  - Surgical intervention may be required.

MICRO-facts

Indications for surgical intervention:
- Age > 60 years.
- Chronic history.
- Relapse on medical treatment.
- Serious co-existing disease.
- Continuous GI bleeding.
- More than 4 units of blood in 24 hours needed.
- Visible ulcer base.
- Clot adherent to ulcer.
- Blood in stomach of unknown origin.

6.7.3 ROCKALL SCORE

- This score is used to identify patients at risk of a poor outcome from GI bleeding. A score of <3 indicates a good outcome is likely, whereas >8 indicates a poor prognosis (Table 6.3).

Table 6.3 The Rockall score

SCORE	0	1	2	3
Age	<60.	60–79.	>80.	
Shock	No shock.	Pulse >100 bpm.	Systolic BP < 100 mmHg.	
Comorbidity	No major comorbidities.		CHD, IHD.	Renal failure, liver failure, metastatic disease.
Diagnosis	Mallory–Weiss tear.	All other diagnoses.	GI malignancy.	
Evidence of bleeding	None.		Blood, adherent clot, bleeding vessel.	

6.8 HOW TO MANAGE ACUTE DYSPHAGIA

- Dysphagia is difficulty in swallowing.
- Odynophagia (painful swallowing) should raise the suspicion of carcinoma.

6.8.1 CAUSES

- Causes of dysphagia may be related to external compression, intrinsic oesophageal disease, motility or neurological disease, or disorders within the mouth or pharynx (Figure 6.10).

6.8.2 DIAGNOSIS

- History is important.
    - Is there progressive dysphagia starting with solid food moving to liquids?
    - Has a food bolus become lodged in a known stricture or tumour?
    - Was it acute—has the patient swallowed a foreign body that has become stuck?
    - Can patient tolerate anything by mouth now?
- Plain chest x-ray (CXR) to demonstrate lesions outside of the oesophagus.
- Barium swallow may demonstrate many compressive diseases, e.g. intrinsic compression, extrinsic compression, pharyngeal pouch, achalasia.
- Upper GI endoscopy is the gold standard for visualisation of the oesophagus, removal of foreign bodies and biopsy of suspicious lesions.
    - There is a risk of perforation, and it should not be performed if a pharyngeal pouch is suspected.
- Manometry and pH monitoring can be useful in achalasia.

General surgery

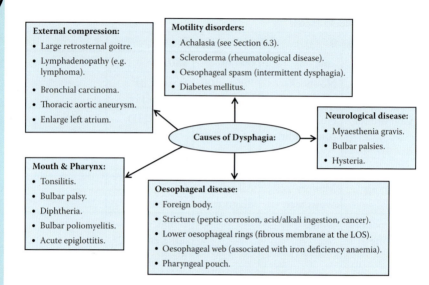

External compression:
- Large retrosternal goitre.
- Lymphadenopathy (e.g. lymphoma).
- Bronchial carcinoma.
- Thoracic aortic aneurysm.
- Enlarge left atrium.

Motility disorders:
- Achalasia (see Section 6.3).
- Scleroderma (rheumatological disease).
- Oesophageal spasm (intermittent dysphagia).
- Diabetes mellitus.

Neurological disease:
- Myaesthenia gravis.
- Bulbar palsies.
- Hysteria.

Causes of Dysphagia:

Mouth & Pharynx:
- Tonsilitis.
- Bulbar palsy.
- Diphtheria.
- Bulbar poliomyelitis.
- Acute epiglottitis.

Oesophageal disease:
- Foreign body.
- Stricture (peptic corrosion, acid/alkali ingestion, cancer).
- Lower oesophageal rings (fibrous membrane at the LOS).
- Oesophageal web (associated with iron deficiency anaemia).
- Pharyngeal pouch.

Figure 6.10 Causes of dysphagia.

- CT scanning will demonstrate extrinsic pathology and will stage the local extent and distal spread of a cancerous lesion.

6.8.3 MANAGEMENT

- Initial management:
    - Ensure there is IV access and maintenance of fluids.
    - If the patient is unable to tolerate anything orally or is at risk of aspiration it may be best to keep him or her nil by mouth (NBM).
        - Absolute dysphagia (i.e. unable to even swallow own saliva) is an emergency and needs immediate intervention to prevent aspiration.
- Further management will depend on the cause.
    - Most patients will require an OGD early in the admission to determine the cause.
    - Many patients admitted acutely with dysphagia are patients with known oesophageal tumours who have a deterioration in symptoms and will often require palliative stenting procedures.

6.9 PEPTIC ULCER DISEASE

6.9.1 DEFINITION

- Mucosal inflammation and acid erosion in the oesophagus, stomach, duodenum.

General surgery

6.9.2 EPIDEMIOLOGY

- Approximately 10–15% of the population will suffer from a duodenal ulcer.
- The incidence of duodenal ulceration is falling; gastric ulcers remain constant.
- Peptic ulcers are relatively rare in developing communities, indicating an environmental influence.

6.9.3 AETIOLOGY

- Peptic ulcers occur where there is both secretion of pepsin and acid. The ulceration is caused by the enzymatic action of pepsin on the mucosa, but this can only occur in the presence of acid. The causes are now well known:
  - Vast majority of ulcers are caused by *Helicobacter pylori*.
    - *H. pylori* is a Gram-negative organism able to survive in the acidic stomach. It has flagella that enable it to move to the mucus layer; it produces urease and has a cell membrane containing hydrogen pumps to prevent acid damage by neutralisation.
  - May occur when there is poor blood supply to the stomach, for example following major surgery, resuscitation or following prolonged stay in intensive care.
  - Rarely, it is caused by Zollinger-Ellison syndrome, which is the presence of a gastrin-secreting tumour. This often causes duodenal ulcers.
  - Other associated factors include:
    - long-term use of NSAIDs and steroids;
    - smoking by reducing mucosal defences and healing;
    - stress;
    - alcohol misuse causing a chronic gastritis.

6.9.4 CLASSIFICATION

- Peptic ulcer disease can be classified by site (duodenal, gastric, oesophageal or Meckel's diverticulum ulcers) and by the modified Johnson classification:
  - Type I: Ulcer along the body of the stomach, most often the lesser curve.
  - Type II: Ulcer in the body in combination with duodenal ulcers. Associated with acid over-secretion.
  - Type III: In the pyloric area within 3 cm of pylorus. Associated with acid over-secretion.
  - Type IV: Proximal gastro-oesophageal ulcer.
  - Type V: Can occur throughout the stomach. Associated with chronic NSAID use (such as aspirin).

General surgery

6.9.5 CLINICAL FEATURES

- The main symptom in peptic ulcer disease is epigastric pain.
  - Radiation to the back suggests a posterior penetrating ulcer.
- Table 6.4 shows signs/symptoms that may allow differentiation between a gastric and duodenal ulcer.

Table 6.4 The differences between gastric and duodenal ulcers.

SYMPTOM/SIGN	GASTRIC ULCER	DUODENAL ULCER
Male:female	3:1	5:1
Age at presentation	50 years	25–30 years
Relationship to eating	Precipitated by food.	Relieved by eating.
Vomiting	Pain relieved by vomiting.	Vomiting is rare.
Cyclical	Not cyclical.	Occurs in cycles lasting about 2 weeks.
Abdominal tenderness	Epigastric.	Epigastric.

6.9.6 DIAGNOSIS

- Gastroscopy is the gold standard diagnostic test. Biopsies should be taken:
  - Gastric carcinomas may present as ulcers.
  - Antral biopsies should be taken for a *Campylobacter*-like organism (CLO) test to identify *H. pylori*.
    - May also be detected by carbon urea breath test or faecal antigen.
- Faecal occult blood is often positive in the presence of an ulcer. This is important in colorectal cancer screening.
- FBC: Bleeding ulcers may cause occult anaemia
- U&E, Ca^{2+}, PO_4 and fasting gastrin levels if hypergastrinaemia is suspected.

6.9.7 MANAGEMENT

- Management may be divided into general measures, medical and surgical management (Figure 6.11).

6.9.8 COMPLICATIONS

Haemorrhage

- Acute bleeding presents with haematemesis or melena.
  - Posterior ulcers may erode into the gastroduodenal artery; lesser curve ulcers may erode into the left gastric artery.
- Bleeding ulcers can be treated at endoscopy with injection of adrenaline or sclerotherapy, diathermy or laser coagulation.

General surgery

General measures:

- Stop smoking, reduce alcohol intake, avoidance of NSAIDs.
- Eradication of *H.pylori* with "Triple therapy".

Triple therapy:

A PPI and 2 antibiotics for 14 days, e.g. metronidazole & clarithromycin (PMC) or amoxicillin & clarithromycin (PAC).

Medical management:

- Antacids provide symptomatic pain relief but are not therapeutic.
- H_2 antagonists (e.g. ranitidine). Histamine promotes release of stomach acid, blocking this reduces ulceration.
- PPIs (e.g. omeprazole). Most effective for symptom control. Prevents acid formation by inhibiting the proton pump.

Surgical management:

- Now rarely necessary due to improved medical therapy.

Indications for surgical intervention:

- Gastric outlet obstruction.
- Failure to respond to maximal medical therapy.
- Emergency (e.g. perforation, bleeding).

Figure 6.11 Management of peptic ulcer disease.

- Surgery may be indicated in high-risk patients or those suffering two rebleeds.
- Immediate surgery may be needed in patients with exsanguinating haemorrhage.
    - A duodenotomy is performed and the bleeding blood vessel is under-run to stop the bleeding. The ulcer is excised and a partial gastrectomy may be required.
- The patient should receive medical therapy following surgery.
- Perforation:
    - Causes severe, constant pain that may be referred to one or both shoulders and is aggravated by movement.
    - There may be generalised peritonitis with marked abdominal rigidity and shallow respiration.
    - Subsequent hypotension, pallor, tachycardia and a mild fever may develop, with eventual progression to shock.
    - Erect chest x-ray will establish the diagnosis in 70% of cases with air under the diaphragm (see above, Figure 6.12).
        - If chest x-ray is uncertain, a CT scan may be used.
        - Plain abdominal x-ray (AXR) may also demonstrate free air by outlining both sides of the bowel wall with air (Rigler's sign).
    - Treatment is with initial resuscitation (cannulation and volume replacement), usually followed by surgical intervention.
        - Surgical closure of the perforation and reinforcement with an omental patch.
        - Some small perforations with little contamination (e.g. following OGD where the stomach is empty) may be managed conservatively with antibiotics, nasogastric (NG) tube and catheterisation, but must be carefully observed for signs of deterioration, which should prompt consideration of surgical intervention.

General surgery

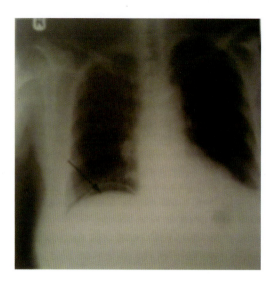

Figure 6.12 Free air visible under the right hemi-diaphragm. (From: *Bailey & Love's Short Practice of Surgery, 26th Edition*, Figure 17.3, p. 376.)

- Mortality of perforation is around 5–10%, due to incorrect diagnosis, delay in treatment or the patient being too ill for operation. The majority of mortality is seen in those 70 years and over.
- Stricture/stenosis of the lumen, important particularly if at the pylorus, as this causes gastric outlet obstruction.
- Potential for malignant change. It is important that whenever a gastric ulcer is seen, a biopsy is taken from the ulcer edge to exclude malignancy.

MICRO-print

Surgical procedures for peptic ulcer disease:

- **Vagotomy:** Vagal stimulation causes acid release. Cutting the vagal nerve also causes gastric paralysis and so a drainage procedure is required (e.g. pyloroplasty or gastrojejunostomy).
- **Highly selective vagotomy:** Aims to only remove vagal stimulation at the area of the parietal cell mass in the body of the stomach, to reduce acid secretion but preserve gastric emptying. Ulcer recurrence rate is higher.
- **Partial gastrectomy:** More historical. Two types: Billroth and Polya. Not used commonly, as side effects are common.

6.10 STOMACH CANCER

> **MICRO-print**
> Most tumours of the stomach are malignant, but occasionally tumours of the stomach may be benign. They may arise from the epithelium, connective tissue or vasculature of the stomach.

6.10.1 EPIDEMIOLOGY

- Gastric cancer is the fourth most common cancer worldwide.
- The incidence is highest in Japan and Chile.
- The peak incidence is 50–70 years of age, with an M:F ratio of 1.8:1.

6.10.2 AETIOLOGY

- Predisposing conditions:
    - Atrophic gastritis. The first step on a pathway of inflammation, metaplasia, dysplasia and carcinoma. It most commonly occurs on the lesser curvature of the stomach.
    - Pernicious anaemia.
    - Previous gastric resection.
    - History of gastric ulceration. Gives rise to 1% of gastric cancers.
- Environmental factors:
    - *H. pylori* infection. This is recognised by the World Health Organisation (WHO) as a class 1 gastric carcinogen; however fewer than 1% of those with *H. pylori* will go on to develop gastric cancer.
    - Low socioeconomic status.
    - Dietary; vegetables and reduced salt and nitrates may be protective.
- Genetic factors:
    - blood group A;
    - associated with alterations in the p53 and APC genes.

6.10.3 PATHOLOGY

- Almost exclusively adenocarcinomas, they occur most often in the antrum.
- Microscopically, there are two subgroups:
    - Intestinal type with cells that grow in clumps. Has a poor prognosis.
    - Diffuse type ('signet ring'). Cells are singular or in small groups and contain large droplets of intracellular mucin.
- Macroscopically there are four appearances (Figure 6.13):
    - malignant ulcer (with raised, everted edges);
    - polypoid tumour (that grows into the lumen of the stomach);
    - colloid tumour (diffuse, gelatinous mass);

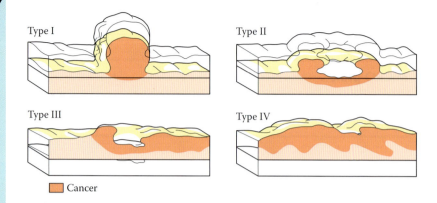

Type I

Type II

Type III

Type IV

■ Cancer

Figure 6.13 Boermann classification of advanced gastric cancer. (From: *Bailey & Love's Short Practice of Surgery, 26th Edition*, Figure 60.28, p. 1069.)

- linitis plastica or 'leather-bottle stomach' (submucosal infiltration causing a rigid, thickened and contracted stomach).
- Metastatic disease:
    - The tumours spread locally to the oesophagus and duodenum, and may infiltrate into other adjacent organs (e.g. liver, transverse colon).
    - The lymph nodes of the lesser curve of the stomach are commonly involved. Mediastinal nodes and thereafter the supraclavicular nodes may be affected (Troisier's sign = enlargement of Virchow's node due to metastases from stomach cancer). The hepatic nodes may also be involved.
    - Haematogenous spread to the liver, lung and bone.
    - The cells may also spread through the abdominal cavity and may cause tumours to develop in the ovaries (Krunkenberg tumours).
    - A gastro-colic fistula may occur that will lead to faecal vomiting.

6.10.4 CLINICAL FEATURES

- 70% present with advanced disease.
- Dyspepsia is the most common symptom.
    - Indistinguishable from that of peptic ulcer disease.
    - The pain may vary in intensity and may be constant and severe.
    - This may radiate to the back, suggesting pancreatic involvement.
- Vomiting, especially if the tumour is obstructing outflow from the stomach.
- As patients often have advanced disease, there is often nausea and weight loss.
- Patients may complain of early satiety.
- Dysphagia may occur if the tumour is in the fundus.

- The tumour may bleed, though frank haematemesis is unusual, and faecal occult blood loss may cause anaemia.
- There is no pattern of symptoms that easily identifies gastric carcinoma.
- On examination, half of patients will have an epigastric mass with abdominal tenderness (this usually indicates that surgical cure will not be possible).
- Patients may have evidence of nodal or distant metastasis.
- Ascites may be present.
- It is the malignancy most commonly associated with dermatomyositis and acanthosis nigricans.

6.10.5 DIAGNOSIS

- Blood tests:
  - FBC may show anaemia.
  - LFTs may be deranged if liver metastases have occurred.
- Gastroscopy allows visualisation and biopsy of lesions. The detection rate of cancer is related to the number of biopsies taken, and it is recommended that 8–10 biopsies be taken around an ulcer. Infiltrative carcinoma may not cause an obvious lesion, and hence the diagnosis may be missed.
  - Linitis plastica will result in a non-distensible stomach at gastroscopy.
- Barium meal may show a filling defect, an ulcer with uneven edges or a thickened rigid stomach in linitis plastica.

6.10.6 STAGING

- CT will demonstrate wall thickening, lymph node involvement, local invasion and hepatic secondaries.
- Ultrasound may also show masses and wall thickening.
- Endoscopic ultrasound will demonstrate the depth of tumour penetration and local invasion. It will also pick up hepatic spread and ascites.
- Laparoscopy may be used to identify peritoneal deposits.
- The tumour, nodes, metastases (TNM) staging system is used in gastric cancer (Table 6.5):
  - T describes how many of the five layers of the stomach wall the tumour has invaded through.

6.10.7 MANAGEMENT

- This is surgical, if the cancer is detected early (T1/2, N0/1), and radical surgery offers the only prospect of cure even when the tumour is small.
  - Surgery may be open or laparoscopic [this may be in the form of laparoscopically assisted digital gastrectomy (LADG)] and may be total or partial.
  - In the UK most patients present too late for the chance of curative surgery.

General surgery

Table 6.5 TNM staging for gastric cancer.

NUMBER	TUMOUR	NODE	METASTASIS
X	Main tumour cannot be assessed.	Regional nodes cannot be assessed.	
0	No tumour found.	No regional lymph nodes found to be involved.	No distant metastases.
In situ	Tumour cells not invaded past the mucosal layer.		
1	Tumour invaded lamina propria or muscularis mucosa.	Involved nodes seen within 3 cm of the primary tumour.	Distant metastases.
	Tumour invaded the submucosal layer.		
2	Tumour invaded into the muscularis propria.	Involved nodes are greater than 3 cm away from primary.	
3	Tumour invaded into the subserosal layer.	Tumour has spread to greater than 15 lymph nodes.	
4	Tumour has invaded through serosa but not into adjacent organs.		
	Tumour has invaded into adjacent organs.		

- Patients undergoing curative procedures should also be considered for D2 lymphadenectomy.
- With any tumour staged at T3 or above curative surgery is not possible; however surgery may be performed with palliative intent.
  - In antral tumours, the tumour may be bypassed by gastrojejunostomy.
  - Palliative gastrectomy is sometimes performed if the patient is suffering from severe problems with nausea, anorexia or vomiting.
  - Stenting may also be used.
  - The number of patients undergoing surgery has reduced due to better staging of the patient, and the 5-year survival rate of those undergoing surgery is now 30%.
    - In Japan where there is better screening and the disease is caught earlier, survival rates are much higher.

- Chemotherapy is used in advanced disease:
  - 5-Fluorouracil appears to be the best agent, though outcome is better when combined with newer agents.
  - Currently being investigated for their use are intraperitoneal chemotherapy and neoadjuvant chemotherapy.

> **MICRO-references**
>
> For more information on chemotherapy for gastric cancer see NICE guidelines TA191, Capecitabine for the treatment of advanced gastric cancer, and TA208, Trastuzumab for the treatment of HER2-positive metastatic gastric cancer.

6.10.8 PROGNOSIS

- The overall prognosis for gastric cancer is only 20%, but this varies with stage.
  - Stage I disease has 80% 5-year survival, but only 1 in 100 patients are found at this stage.
  - 80% of patients are diagnosed with stage IV disease, and this carries a 5-year survival outcome of 5%.
  - In trials, chemotherapy has been found to extend 5-year survival to 36%.

> **MICRO-case**
>
> A 55-year-old male presents with a 2-month history of lethargy and malaise. His only regular medication is omeprazole, which was started 4 months earlier for indigestion.
>
> On examination he appears slightly pale, but there are no other clinical signs to note. An FBC and LFT revealed the following:
>
> | | | | |
> |---|---|---|---|
> | Hb | 8 g/dL | Bilirubin | 15 µmol/L |
> | WCC | 10×10^9/L | ALT | 30 U/L |
> | Plt | 200×10^9/L | AST | 26 U/L |
> | MVC | 68 fL | ALP | 56 U/L |
>
> He is referred for upper and lower GI endoscopies. An OGD reveals a large ulcer in the body of the stomach with heaped edges and a CLO was positive. Biopsies of the ulcer edge reveal adenocarcinoma. He proceeds to have full staging investigations.
>
> **Learning points:**
> - The presenting features of gastric carcinoma are non-specific and often may be indistinguishable from a simple peptic ulcer.
> - Patients presenting with dyspepsia after the age of 50 should be thoroughly investigated.
> - Any male or post-menopausal women with anaemia of unknown origin should undergo investigation to rule out a sinister cause.

General surgery

6.11 INTESTINAL ISCHAEMIA

6.11.1 AETIOLOGY

- Acute mesenteric ischaemia may be due to arterial, venous or mixed causes.
  - Arterial:
    - Acute occlusion of the superior mesenteric artery (SMA) is the commonest cause of small bowel ischaemia and may be:
    - embolic (usually from the heart after MI or AF);
    - thrombotic (due to dislodgement of atherosclerotic plaque).
  - Venous:
    - portal vein thrombosis;
    - low-flow states (e.g. hypotension, dehydration, following MI);
    - hypercoagulable states (protein C or S deficiency, factor V Leiden).
  - Mixed:
    - internal mesenteric hernia;
    - bowel-containing incarcerated abdominal wall hernia.
- Chronic mesenteric ischaemia is due to atherosclerotic plaques and clinically manifests in the watershed area (the splenic flexure) where the territories of the SMA and IMA meet.

6.11.2 CLINICAL FEATURES

- Acute SMA occlusion presents as an acute abdomen and is a surgical emergency.
  - Severe non-specific abdominal pain of sudden onset.
    - Pain is typically 'out of proportion' to the clinical findings.
  - The abdomen may initially remain soft with subsequent development of peritonitis due to transmural necrosis and translocation of bacteria.
  - Raised heart rate, cold extremities and tachypnoea with rapid progression to shock.
  - There may be vomiting and diarrhoea.
  - The patient may be in fast AF.
- Chronic ischaemia presents more insidiously:
  - Post-prandial abdominal pain with associated weight loss as the patient becomes afraid of eating.
  - There may be features of ischaemic colitis (e.g. PR bleeding) or strictures.
  - An abdominal bruit may be present in severe stenosis.

6.11.3 DIAGNOSIS

- General investigations:
  - raised WCC;
  - metabolic acidosis with a raised lactate on ABG;
  - AF or tachycardia on ECG.

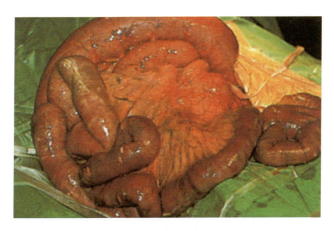

Figure 6.14 Acute mesenteric ischaemia with discoloured loops of small intestine. (From: *Illustrated Clinical Anatomy, 2nd ed.*, Figure 3.17, p. 97.)

- CT scanning may reveal gas in the bowel wall or portal system. It may also demonstrate the cause (such as cut-off of arterial contrast at the SMA or the presence of an internal hernia).
- Mesenteric angiography may differentiate between embolic, thrombotic or non-occlusive ischaemia.
- The diagnosis may be confirmed on diagnostic laparotomy, which should not be delayed if acute small bowel infarction is suspected (Figure 6.14).

6.11.4 MANAGEMENT

- Urgent resuscitation using the ABCDE approach:
    - Wide-bore cannulas, aggressive intravenous fluids, antibiotics and oxygen therapy.
    - Involve senior surgeons and anaesthetists early.
- Treat fast AF.
- The mainstay of therapy is surgical resection of necrotic bowel at laparotomy, and this should be performed urgently to reduce mortality.
    - Stoma formation is performed, as the risk of anastamotic breakdown is high due to poor blood flow.
    - There is an indication for a 're-look' laparotomy after 24 hours to assess the viability of remaining bowel that wasn't frankly necrotic at first look.
    - Patients should be managed in the critical care setting post-operatively.
- Restoration of blood flow to the bowel may be possible:
    - anticoagulation;
    - vasodilators;
    - embolectomy;

General surgery

- angioplasty (in chronic cases);
- aorto-mesenteric bypass procedures (rarely performed).

6.11.5 PROGNOSIS

- Mortality from acute small bowel infarction is 60–90%.
- Delay in diagnosis increases this risk.

6.12 SMALL BOWEL OBSTRUCTION

6.12.1 Aetiology

- Mechanical obstruction is caused by a physical blockage.
  - May be complete or incomplete.
- Functional obstruction refers to the paralysis of intestinal transit.
  - Also known as paralytic ileus, pseudo-obstruction.
  - Usually due to over-activity of the sympathetic nervous system.

6.12.2 PATHOLOGY

- In mechanical obstruction, the bowel distal to the obstruction rapidly empties and collapses. The proximal bowel distends and dilates with gas (most of which is swallowed air) and intestinal secretions.
  - Fluid sequestration within the bowel lumen results in depletion of the extracellular fluid with subsequent dehydration and electrolyte imbalance. This is compounded by the accompanying vomiting.
- There is increased peristalsis in an attempt to overcome the obstruction, which results in the abdominal colic.
- As the bowel wall distends, there is venous congestion, followed by impaired arterial supply leading to patchy mucosal necrosis and transmural translocation of bacteria across the wall with consequent peritonitis.
- Perforation may eventually be the result in severe cases, from either wall distension or necrosis at the site of obstruction.

MICRO-facts

Causes of mechanical small bowel obstruction:
- **In the lumen:** Bezoars, gallstone 'ileus', food bolus, parasites, intussusception.
- **In the wall:** Congenital atresia, Crohn's disease, tumours.
- **Outside the wall:** Hernia (internal or external), adhesions, congenital bands, volvulus.

General surgery

6.12.3 CLINICAL FEATURES

- There are four cardinal features of intestinal obstruction:
  - colicky abdominal pain;
  - abdominal distension;
  - absolute constipation (i.e. no passage of flatus or stools);
  - vomiting.
- Depending on the level of obstruction, different features will predominate:
  - High obstruction (e.g. gastric outlet obstruction) results in early vomiting, but there will not be abdominal distension.
  - Lower-level obstruction (e.g. terminal ileal Crohn's) results in more distension and later vomiting.
  - N.B. In large bowel obstruction absolute constipation would be the predominant feature and vomiting would be a late sign.
- Search for signs suggesting an obvious cause, e.g.:
  - irreducible hernia;
  - scars suggesting previous surgery with possible adhesional origin.

6.12.4 DIAGNOSIS

Biochemistry

- FBC: ↑ WCC suggests sepsis and possible strangulation.
- U&E: Monitor for electrolyte disturbances and dehydration.
- ABG: Development of metabolic acidosis is a poor prognostic sign.
  - Rising lactate suggests strangulation and ischaemia.

Imaging

- AXR is key diagnostic tool (Figure 6.15).
- Erect CXR may be useful if associated perforation is suspected.
- CT scan may be useful to distinguish the cause.

Diagnostic laparotomy

- The exact cause may not be found until surgery is performed.

6.12.5 MANAGEMENT

- Initial conservative management should be initiated early (prior to possible surgery):
  - Good intravenous access with IV fluids.
  - Nasogastric (NG) tube with regular repeated aspiration.
  - Monitoring of fluid balance (urinary catheter, CVP line may be required).

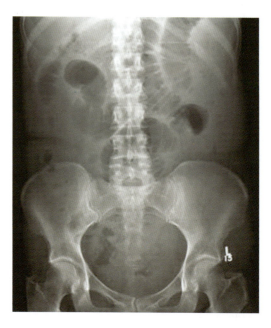

Figure 6.15 Supine abdominal x-ray showing multiple dilated small bowel loops, classical of small bowel obstruction. (From: *Bailey & Love's Short Practice of Surgery, 26th Edition*, Figure 13.1, p. 173.)

- Close observation for deterioration over the first 24 hours.
  - A good outcome from conservative therapy is suggested by reduction of abdominal pain, reduced NG aspirates, lessening of abdominal distension and the passage of flatus.
  - A trial of conservative treatment is often successful in patients with adhesional obstruction.
    - These patients should have regular reviews to ensure there is no clinical deterioration that would mandate surgical intervention.
- Urgent surgery should be considered in all cases where there is evidence of ischaemia or impending perforation.
  - Abdominal tenderness is particularly important, and development of peritonism should prompt review and consideration of surgical intervention.
  - Patients with irreducible hernias or 'virgin' abdomens usually require operative intervention early.
- Early reinstatement of nutrition is important, with enteral feeding preferred where tolerated.

6.12.6 COMPLICATIONS

- Necrosis, perforation, peritonitis, death.
- Dehydration, electrolyte disturbances, AF.

6.12.7 PROGNOSIS

- With early treatment the prognosis is good.

MICRO-case

A 75-year-old women presents with a 4-day history of colicky, central abdominal pain and vomiting green-brown fluid. She has also not opened her bowels for a couple of days.

On examination she has dry mucous membranes. Her abdomen is distended, tympanic but soft, and there is a Pfannensteil scar from surgery performed 30 years ago. Digital rectal examination reveals an empty, collapsed rectum. Her HR is 110 bpm, BP is 100/60 mmHg, RR is 20/min and she is apyrexial. A plain AXR reveals central dilated loops of small bowel.

You gain IV access, administer an IV bolus and prescribe an analgesic and anti-emetic. You proceed to place an NG tube and urinary catheter. Her blood tests and ABG reveal the following:

Hb	15.6 g/dL	WCC	10.5×10^9/L
Na	132 mmol/L	K	3.2 mmol/L
Cr	154 mmol/L	u	8.9 mmol/L
ABG	Metabolic acidosis with a raised lactate		

Learning points:

- This woman has small bowel obstruction, probably secondary to adhesions from her previous gynaecological surgery—even though this was many years ago and she has never had similar problems.
- She should be resuscitated with IV fluids and monitored closely, as she may settle with conservative treatment only.
- A CT scan may help confirm the diagnosis of adhesional aetiology.
- If there are any signs of deterioration, surgical intervention should be considered.

6.13 SMALL BOWEL TUMOURS

- Small bowel malignancies account for less than 2% of all GI malignancies and usually present at an advanced stage.
- Diagnosis is aided by double-contrast small bowel follow-through, CT scanning and capsule endoscopy.

6.13.1 PEUTZ-JEGHERS HAMARTOMA

- Familial syndrome where there are multiple intestinal polyps and mucosal melanin spots.
- Polyps may be up to 3 cm and cause intussusception or bleeding.
- They are benign and therefore only removed if symptomatic.

6.13.2 ADENOMA

- May be associated with familial adenomatous polyposis (FAP).
- Very rarely associated with malignant change in high-grade villous form.

6.13.3 GASTROINTESTINAL STROMAL TUMOUR (GIST)

- Rare mesenchymal tumours of the GI tract.
  - Account for less than 1% of all primary neoplasms.
- Different subtypes with varying malignant potential.
- Initial management is with surgical resection.
  - Recurrent disease may be managed with a combination of chemotherapy, further resection, radiofrequency ablation and imatinib mesylate therapy.

6.13.4 ADENOCARCINOMA

- Most common in the duodenum, least common in the ileum.
- FAP, Crohn's disease and coeliac disease are risk factors.
- Symptoms are vague and non-specific.
- They are usually diagnosed late.
- Treatment is with en bloc resection—taking adjacent affected organs with the small bowel.
- Prognosis is usually 10–20% at 5 years due to late presentation.

6.13.5 CARCINOID (NEUROENDOCRINE TUMOURS)

- Most common in the appendix and terminal ileum.
- Capable of secreting neuroendocrine substances (e.g. 5-hydroxytryptamine).
- Metastases to lymph nodes and liver are common.
- Carcinoid syndrome is caused by metastasis of carcinoid tumours to the liver.
  - Symptoms are of severe facial flushing, diarrhoea and asthma attacks.
- Treatment is surgical resection.

6.13.6 LYMPHOMA

- Most common in the ileum.
- Primary small bowel lymphoma is treated by surgical resection.
- Secondary small bowel lymphoma is treated in the traditional way with chemotherapy.

General surgery

7 Colorectal

7.1 ANATOMY OF THE BOWEL

- The colon is the last part of the digestive system. It begins at the ileocolic junction and is divided into caecum, ascending colon, transverse colon, descending colon, sigmoid colon and rectum.
- Its main function is the absorption of water, sodium and some fat-soluble vitamins (i.e. vitamin K, vitamin B_{12}, thiamine and riboflavin) from faecal matter, before excreting the indigestible food matter from the body via the anus.
- Its blood supply is from the superior and inferior mesenteric arteries (Figures 7.1 and 7.2), as well as the middle and inferior rectal arteries.

7.2 APPENDICITIS

7.2.1 EPIDEMIOLOGY

- Commonest cause of an acute abdomen and surgical admission in the UK.
- Approximately one in seven people will have an appendicectomy.
- It most commonly occurs between 10 and 20 years; it is rare under 3 years of age.

7.2.2 PATHOLOGY

- The aetiology is unknown but inflammation may be precipitated by faecoliths, hyperplasia of lymphoid tissue, foreign bodies or rarely tumours of the caecum or carcinoid tumours of the appendix (Figure 7.3).

7.2.3 CLINICAL FEATURES

Abdominal pain
- Initially vague, colicky central abdominal pain.
  - Visceral pain caused by luminal obstruction of the appendix and stretch of the visceral peritoneum.
- Localising to the right iliac fossa and becoming constant.
  - The pain changes as the parietal peritoneum becomes involved.

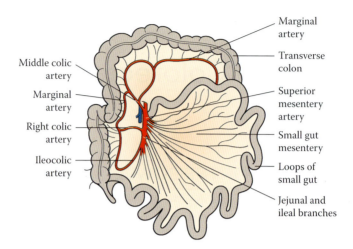

Figure 7.1 Superior mesenteric artery and its branches. (From: *Illustrated Clinical Anatomy*, 2nd *Edition.*, Figure 6.15, p. 96.)

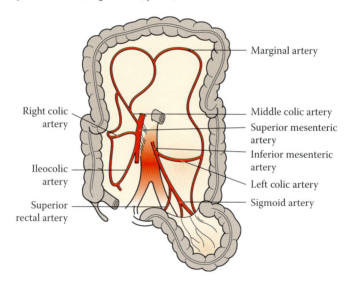

Figure 7.2 Superior and inferior mesenteric arterial supply of the large intestine. (From: *Illustrated Clinical Anatomy, 2nd Edition.*, Figure 6.16, p. 96.)

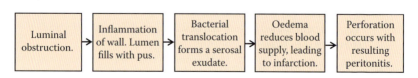

| Luminal obstruction. | → | Inflammation of wall. Lumen fills with pus. | → | Bacterial translocation forms a serosal exudate. | → | Oedema reduces blood supply, leading to infarction. | → | Perforation occurs with resulting peritonitis. |

Figure 7.3 Pathological process of acute appendicitis.

- Usually accompanied by a low-grade fever, nausea, vomiting and anorexia.
- The appendix position varies and can result in different symptoms; for example a pelvic appendix may cause urinary symptoms or diarrhoea.
- On examination there may be general signs of sepsis:
  - Usually a low-grade pyrexia initially, which may spike up to 38–39°C in the presence of perforation or abscess formation.
  - There may be tachycardia, flushing and evidence of dehydration.

Abdominal examination

- Tenderness over McBurney's point is the usual feature.
  - There may also be signs of peritoneal inflammation, including:
    - Guarding, tenderness on percussion, pain on coughing or other movement.
  - Signs of generalised peritonitis may develop as the illness progresses with abdominal rigidity.
- Rovsing's sign: Pain is felt in the RIF when pressure is applied to the LIF.
  - There must also be RIF tenderness for this sign to be positive.
- Psoas sign: The patient keeps his or her hip in flexion to relieve his or her pain.
  - The appendix is anatomically adjacent to the psoas muscle, which is involved in hip flexion.
- PR examination may reveal tenderness anterolaterally on the right.

MICRO-facts

McBurney's point is a point 2/3 of the way between the umbilicus and the right anterior superior iliac spine, and overlies the usual location of the appendix base.

7.2.4 DIAGNOSIS

- The diagnosis of appendicitis is a clinical one; however there are some tests that may be useful, particularly where the diagnosis is not clear-cut. These include:
  - The performance of a full blood count (FBC) can be useful to determine whether or not the patient has a leucocytosis.
  - A urinalysis to exclude urinary tract infection.
    - Although appendicitis may cause a haematuria or pyuria with associated urinary symptoms.
  - A pregnancy test in women of child-bearing age is mandatory to rule out an ectopic pregnancy.
  - An ultrasound scan (USS) in women can be useful where the diagnosis of appendicitis is in doubt to exclude tubo-ovarian pathology as the cause of RIF pain.

- A computed tomography (CT) scan can be useful to confirm the diagnosis, especially in the elderly where a caecal tumour may be causative, or in the obese where examination is difficult.
- Diagnostic laparoscopy allows immediate treatment if appendicitis is confirmed.
- Urea and electrolytes (U&E) should also be performed to assess hydration status.
- Remember to ask about previous abdominal surgeries (including right hemicolectomy), as it is embarrassing to quote appendicitis as a cause of RIF pain if the patient has already had the appendix removed!

7.2.5 MANAGEMENT

- Patients are often dehydrated at presentation and so require fluid resuscitation. IV fluids should be continued whilst the patient remains starved for theatre.

Open appendicectomy

- Usually performed in children.
- A Lanz incision (centred on McBurney's point; see Figure 1.5) is used for the best cosmetic result.
- If the appendix is found to be perforated or gangrenous, then peritoneal lavage is performed to remove any pus or contamination.
- Most patients can be discharged on the second or third day post-operatively.

Laparoscopic appendicectomy

- Improves diagnostic accuracy and minimises negative appendicectomy rates.
  - It is indicated in patients who are unwell but there is question as to the diagnosis, and is particularly indicated in young women.
  - It is useful in the obese where wound infections are more common and laparoscopic procedures have lower wound infection rates.
- There is now evidence to suggest that laparoscopic appendicectomy should be performed where expertise is available for this to be done.
- Laparoscopy has decreased length of stay in hospital, faster return to normal diet and activities and better post-operative pain.
- If the patient presents late (usually after several days of symptoms) with a palpable appendix mass, he or she requires CT scanning to determine whether there is an associated appendix abscess or a perforated caecal tumour.
  - The initial management of an appendix abscess is conservative with IV fluids, antibiotics and observation. They may require radiological drainage.
  - If there is deterioration, or frank perforation, surgery may still be required.

7.2.6 COMPLICATIONS

- Abscess formation; peri-appendicular, pelvic or sub-hepatic.
- Post-operative collection or abscess.
- Appendix stump blowout, leading to peritonitis.
- Wound problems, including infection or haematoma.
- Intestinal obstruction due to adhesion formation within the abdomen.
- Patients with a perforated appendix may occasionally need admission to intensive treatment unit (ITU).

> **MICRO-reference**
> Sauerland S, Lefering R, Neugebauer EAM. Laparoscopic versus open surgery for suspected appendicitis. *Cochrane Database of Systematic Reviews* 2004; 4: art. no.: CD001546. DOI: 10.1002/14651858.CD001546.pub2.

7.3 HOW TO MANAGE A CASE OF SUSPECTED APPENDICITIS

7.3.1 IMMEDIATE MANAGEMENT

- Patients should be kept nil by mouth for surgery.
- Prescribe IV fluids, as dehydration is likely (e.g. normal saline or Hartmann's).
- Ensure adequate analgesia is prescribed.
- IV antibiotics should be prescribed if the patient is septic or when a diagnosis of appendicitis has been made and the patient is waiting for theatre.
    - Broad-spectrum antibiotics, e.g. cefuroxime and metronidazole, are commonly used to cover gastrointestinal (GI) tract organisms.
- Appropriate blood tests (e.g. U&E, group and save), ECG and chest x-ray (CXR) should be performed depending on age and comorbidities, prior to theatre and a general anaesthetic (see Section 1.2).
- As diagnosis of appendicitis is mostly clinical, and if initial conservative management is undertaken, regular review is necessary to identify early deterioration, in which case operative intervention should be expedited.
- In acute appendicitis urgent removal of the appendix is the definitive treatment, rather than antibiotics.
    - Only in the case of an appendix mass, abscess or severe comorbidity precluding anaesthesia, should conservative management and delayed operation be considered.

General surgery

> **MICRO-case**
>
> A 25-year-old female who is 30 weeks pregnant presents to the obstetric unit with abdominal pain that started 8 hours ago. It was initially generalised and intermittent but has now worsened and become constant, localised to the right flank. Foetal movements have also become painful.
>
> Her temperature is 37.8°C and she is tender in the right abdomen, though examination is difficult due to her gravid uterus. Her WCC is 13.5×10^9/L. An ultrasound reveals an inflamed appendix in the right flank.
>
> **Learning points:**
> - Pregnant women have the same risk of appendicitis as non-pregnant women of the same age.
> - As pregnancy progresses, the pain is usually not in the RIF as the uterus pushes the colon upward in the abdomen, making it a difficult diagnosis to make in pregnancy.
> - Early diagnosis and an open operation (with a modified incision) are the best management in the third trimester.

7.4 INFLAMMATORY BOWEL DISEASE

- Differentiating features of Crohn's disease and ulcerative colitis are shown in Table 7.1.

7.5 CROHN'S DISEASE

7.5.1 DEFINITION

- Non-specific chronic granulomatous inflammatory condition affecting any part of the GI tract.

> **MICRO-facts**
>
> Crohn's disease is also known as **terminal ileitis**, as it was first described in the terminal ileum by Crohn. This is a misnomer since pure ileitis occurs in 20% of Crohn's cases.

7.5.2 PATHOLOGY

- Transmural inflammation and ulceration that may lead to abscess formation and fistulae into adjacent visceral structures.
- Submucosal oedema leads to thickening of the wall.

Table 7.1 Epidemiology, aetiology, distribution and prognosis of Crohn's disease and ulcerative colitis.

CHARACTERISTIC	CROHN'S DISEASE	ULCERATIVE COLITIS (UC)
Epidemiology	Incidence = 145 per 100,000. More common in the West. Higher risk in Ashkenazi Jewish populations. M:F = M < F. Mean age of onset = 26 years.	Incidence = 243 per 100,000. More common in the West. Higher risk in Ashkenazi Jewish populations. M:F = M > F. Mean age of onset = 34 years.
Aetiology	Unknown. Association with HLA-B27. More common in smokers. Familial predisposition— up to 40% risk of developing if 1 of 3 mutations of CARD15 gene.	Unknown. Association with HLA-B27. More common in non-smokers. Familial predisposition—gene involved unclear.
Distribution	Anywhere in GI tract. Small bowel only in 50%. Terminal ileum in 50%. Large bowel only in 20%. Small and large bowel in 30%. May just have isolated perianal Crohn's.	From rectum more proximally (occasional rectal sparing). Proctitis. Left-sided colitis (to splenic flexure). Pancolitis. 'Backwash ileitis' may occur.
Prognosis	50% will require surgery within 10 years. 70–80% will require surgery in their lifetime. 75% will be able to go back to work within 1 year.	50% will have a relapse once a year. 20–30% with pancolitis will need a colectomy. 90% will be able to go back to work within 1 year. Surgery can be curative.

General surgery

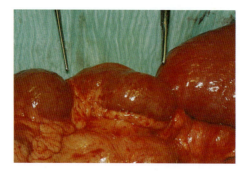

Figure 7.4 Small bowel strictures in Crohn's disease. (From: *Bailey & Love's Short Practice of Surgery, 26th Edition.*)

- Marked fibrosis of wall from long-standing inflammation leads to stricture formation (Figure 7.4).
- Cobblestone appearance of wall due to ulceration and fissuring.
- Skip lesions—areas of 'normal' mucosa between discrete patches of inflammation.
- Fat wrapping—mesenteric fat envelopment of bowel.
- Presence of non-caseating granulomas with multi-nucleate giant cells.

7.5.3 CLINICAL FEATURES

- Clinical features of Crohn's disease are best thought of as those arising from the GI tract, those arising from systemic upset and those due to the extra-GI manifestations of the disease (see Table 7.2 and Figure 7.5).

Table 7.2 Extra-gastrointestinal manifestation (EIM) of Crohn's disease and ulcerative colitis.

	CROHN'S DISEASE	ULCERATIVE COLITIS
Joints	Large joint arthritis.* Ankylosing spondylitis.	Large joint arthritis.* Ankylosing spondylitis.
Skin	Pyoderma gangrenosum.* Erythema nodosum.*	Pyoderma gangrenosum.* Erythema nodosum.*
Eyes	Uveitis.* Episcleritis.* Conjunctivitis.*	Uveitis.* Episcleritis.* Conjunctivitis.*
Liver	Cirrhosis. Fatty liver. Gallstones.	Cirrhosis. Fatty liver. Primary sclerosing cholangitis. Pericholangitis.
Other	Renal oxalate stones.	Venous thrombosis.

* Denotes EIMs that are related to disease activity.

> # MICRO-facts
> Crohn's may present acutely with RIF pain mimicking acute appendicitis.

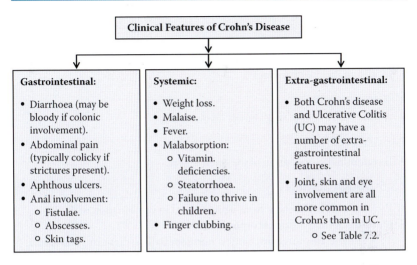

Figure 7.5 Clinical features of Crohn's.

7.5.4 INVESTIGATIONS

FBC
- Anaemia of chronic disease (i.e. normocytic, normochromic).
- Anaemia due to iron deficiency from GI bleeding.
- ↑ white cell count (WCC).

LFT
- ↓ Serum albumin.

Raised ESR and CRP

Stool
- MC&S to rule out infective cause for diarrhoea.
- Faecal calprotectin (confirms presence of inflammatory bowel disease (IBD)).

Barium enema or small bowel follow-through
- Deep ulceration of bowel wall ('rose thorn' appearance).
- Narrow lumen of terminal ileum (secondary to strictures).
- Skin lesions.

- Cobble-stoning.
- Fistulae.

Colonoscopy

- To assess colonic involvement and obtain terminal ileal biopsies.

Indium-labelled leucocyte scan

- Radioactive labelling of leucocytes to determine extent of disease (by localising their aggregation).

MRI enteroclysis

- Allows assessment of small bowel involvement.

Capsule endoscopy

- Intraluminal visualisation of the small bowel.

7.5.5 MANAGEMENT

- Patients with IBD benefit from being treated in combination with a multi-disciplinary team incorporating:
  - Physicians, surgeons, clinical nurse specialists, dieticians and stoma nurses.

General measures

- Smoking cessation can lead to <65% reduction in relapse rate.
- Nutritional supplements.
- Iron supplementation in chronic cases.
- Use of anti-diarrhoeal agents, e.g. codeine and loperamide.

Mainstay of management is medical (see Figure 7.6)

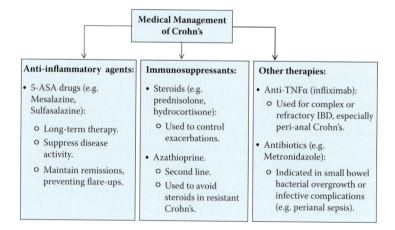

Figure 7.6 Medical management of Crohn's disease.

Surgical management

- Indications:
  - Failure to respond to medical management.
  - Growth retardation in children.
  - Acute complications, e.g. obstruction, perforation, abscesses, enterocutaneous fistulae.
  - Defunctioning of severe perianal disease (e.g., 'watering can perineum').
  - Stricturoplasty in small bowel strictures.
- Aim to resect as little of the bowel as possible as recurrence occurs in approximately 50%.

7.6 ULCERATIVE COLITIS

7.6.1 DEFINITION

- Chronic inflammatory condition of the large bowel only.

7.6.2 PATHOLOGY

- Extensive superficial irregular ulceration of the mucosa.
- Mucosal oedema.
- Continuous inflammation, i.e. no skip lesions.
- Crypt abscesses.
- Formation of pseudopolyps—islands of regenerating mucosa in between areas of ulceration.
- Chronic inflammatory infiltrate.
- Depletion of goblet cells.

MICRO-facts

Clinical features vary according to disease extent, but in general the more proximal the disease, the more systemic the features.

7.6.3 CLINICAL FEATURES

- As with Crohn's disease, the clinical features of ulcerative colitis (UC) can be divided into those arising from the GI tract, those arising from systemic upset and those due to the extra-GI manifestations of the disease (see Figure 7.7).

General surgery

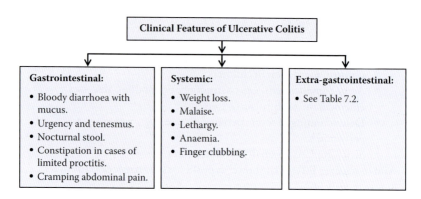

Figure 7.7 Clinical features of UC.

7.6.4 INVESTIGATIONS

FBC
- Microcytic anaemia secondary to iron deficiency.
- ↑ WCC.

LFT
- ↓ Serum albumin.

Raised ESR and CRP
- Useful for disease monitoring.

Stool MC&S
- To rule out an infective cause for diarrhoea.

Faecal calprotectin
- Diagnostic for IBD.

AXR
- In acute exacerbations, may be used to rule out perforation or colonic dilatation. It may also show 'thumbprinting' in acutely inflamed and oedematous bowel.

Barium enema
- In long-standing disease may show loss of haustration ('lead pipe'/'drain pipe' colon).

Lower GI endoscopy
- To confirm diagnosis (biopsy) and determine extent of disease.
- Shows grossly inflamed friable mucosa with contact bleeding (Figure 7.8).
- Often granular appearance of mucosa.

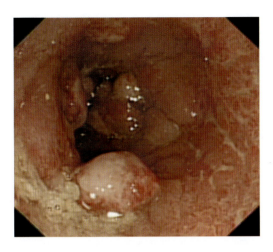

Figure 7.8 Colitis as seen on lower GI endoscopy. (From: *Browse's Introduction to the Investigation and Management of Surgical Disease*, Fig. 19.4, p. 478.)

7.6.5 MANAGEMENT

- Depends on severity of attacks.

General measures

- Anti-diarrhoeal agents, e.g. loperamide, codeine.
  - Should not be used in acute attacks, as can precipitate toxic dilatation.
- Replace lost nutrients, e.g. iron and protein.
- IV fluids and total parenteral nutrition (TPN) used in acute flares to allow bowel rest.

Medical therapy

- 5-ASA (e.g. mesalazine, sulphasalazine):
  - Long-term anti-inflammatory agents used to maintain remission.
  - Topical—as suppositories for proctitis or foam enemas if more proximal.
  - Oral for more extensive disease.
- Steroids:
  - Used to control exacerbations of colitis.
  - Topical or oral depending on extent of disease.
  - Should not be used long term—if unable to withdraw steroid therapy, then surgical management is indicated.
- Azathioprine:
  - Immunosuppressant agent for acute UC.

- Cyclosporin A:
  - Second-line immunosuppressant for acute UC.
  - Can be given IV or as an enema.

Surgical management (see Figure 7.9)

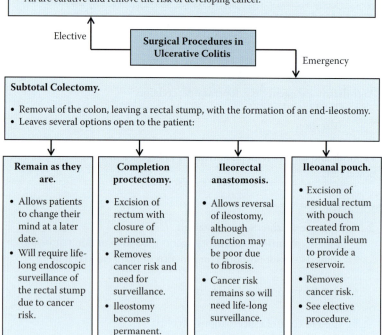

Panproctocolectomy: excision of colon and rectum.

- With a permanent ileostomy.
  - Not reversible as the perineum is closed.
- With an ileoanal anastomosis.
  - Function may be poor due to high quantities of liquid stool without the rectal reservoir.
- With ileoanal pouch (+/– loop ileostomy).
  - Creation of reservoir pouch from terminal ileum.
  - May avoid the need for a permanent ileostomy.
  - May be performed with a covering ileostomy to protect the pouch that can be reversed in a second procedure.
  - Technically more demanding.
  - Complications: pouch failure (3%), leakage, stenosis, pouchitis (15%).
- All are curative and remove the risk of developing cancer.

Elective

Surgical Procedures in Ulcerative Colitis

Emergency

Subtotal Colectomy.

- Removal of the colon, leaving a rectal stump, with the formation of an end-ileostomy.
- Leaves several options open to the patient:

Remain as they are.	**Completion proctectomy.**	**Ileorectal anastomosis.**	**Ileoanal pouch.**
• Allows patients to change their mind at a later date. • Will require life-long endoscopic surveillance of the rectal stump due to cancer risk.	• Excision of rectum with closure of perineum. • Removes cancer risk and need for surveillance. • Ileostomy becomes permanent.	• Allows reversal of ileostomy, although function may be poor due to fibrosis. • Cancer risk remains so will need life-long surveillance.	• Excision of residual rectum with pouch created from terminal ileum to provide a reservoir. • Removes cancer risk. • See elective procedure.

Figure 7.9 Surgical management of ulcerative colitis.

General surgery

MICRO-facts

Indications for surgery in UC:
- Elective:
  - Failure to respond to medical management.
  - Growth retardation in children.
  - Recurrent acute on chronic episodes.
  - Development of dysplasia/carcinoma.
- Emergency:
  - For complications of acute exacerbations (Figure 7.10):
    - Toxic dilatation (Figure 7.11).
    - Perforation.
    - Haemorrhage.

Management of acute severe colitis

- This is a medical emergency.
- Send blood for FBC, U&E, LFT, glucose, CRP, cross-match and haematinics.
- Important to send stool MC&S (especially *Clostridium difficile* toxin assay), as hard to distinguish from infective colitis.
- If the patient is stable, flexible sigmoidoscopy will confirm the diagnosis and demonstrate the extent.
- IV fluid with electrolyte replacement.
- If Hb < 10 g/dL, consider transfusion.

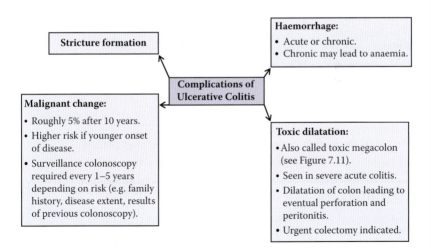

Figure 7.10 Complications of ulcerative colitis.

General surgery

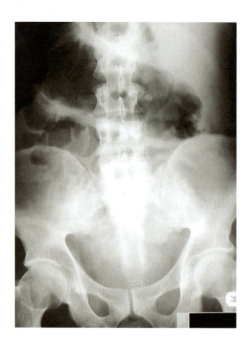

Figure 7.11 A supine abdominal radiograph showing toxic megacolon (the transverse colon is dilated to 7 cm and shows no haustral folds). (From: *Bailey & Love's Short Practice of Surgery, 26th Edition*, Figure 69.3, p. 1147.)

- Give antibiotics in patients with complications (such as toxic megacolon or perforation).
- Subcutaneous heparin to reduce risk of thromboembolism.
- Management should be on the medical ward, as initial treatment is with IV corticosteroids. There should be close liaison with the surgical team.
- If no improvement within 3 days:
  - IV cyclosporin 2 mg/kg/day.
- If no improvement within 4–7 days:
  - Colectomy is recommended—review by the surgical team.

MICRO-facts

Truelove and Witts' criteria for acute severe colitis:
- ≥6 bloody stools per day.
- HR > 90 bpm.
- Temperature > 37.8°C.
- Hb ≤ 10.5 g/dL.
- ESR > 30 mm/hour.

7.7 ISCHAEMIC COLITIS

7.7.1 AETIOLOGY

- Occlusion of inferior mesenteric artery, e.g. by thromboembolism, or acute-on-chronic due to atherosclerosis of the inferior mesenteric artery (IMA) or superior mesenteric artery (SMA).
- Usually in upper left colon—known as the 'watershed' area, it is where the territories of the SMA and IMA meet.

7.7.2 CLINICAL FEATURES

- Abdominal pain.
- Bloody diarrhoea.
- Fever.
- Leucocytosis.

7.7.3 MANAGEMENT

- Supportive as usually resolves spontaneously.
- Broad-spectrum antibiotics.
- Anticoagulation if thromboembolism.
- May progress to acute severe colitis requiring subtotal colectomy.

7.8 INFECTIVE COLITIS

7.8.1 AETIOLOGY

Pseudomembranous colitis

- Infection with *Clostridium difficile*.
- Associated with use of third-generation cephalosporins, co-amoxiclav, and ciprofloxacin.
- Antibiotic reduces the normal gut flora, permitting overgrowth of pathogens.

Other organisms

- E.g. *Escherichia coli* and *Shigella dysenteriae*.

7.8.2 CLINICAL FEATURES

- Diarrhoea.
  - The diarrhoea of pseudomembranous colitis is usually green-coloured and foul-smelling.
- Abdominal pain.
- History of recent antibiotic use (pseudomembranous colitis).
- May be history of foreign travel of contact with other cases.

General surgery

7.8.3 INVESTIGATIONS

- Stool MC&S to identify organism.
- *Clostridium difficile* toxin assay.
- Endoluminal visualisation of pseudomembranes on mucosa.

7.8.4 MANAGEMENT

- Supportive, i.e. fluids with electrolyte replacement.
- Probiotics to replace intraluminal flora.
- Faecal transplantation.
    - Donor needs to be a close family member so he or she shares the same bacterial flora.

Antibiotics

- Vancomycin PO/metronidazole IV in pseudomembranous colitis.
- Other forms of infective colitis will only require antibiotics if severe—base drug choice on results of stool culture.

Surgical

- Sub-total colectomy may rarely be indicated in severe, non-responsive cases.
- Emergency colectomy may also be required in cases of toxic megacolon that result in perforation.

7.9 IRRITABLE BOWEL SYNDROME

- Irritable bowel syndrome (IBS) is a common, functional bowel disorder of unknown aetiology:
    - Prevalence of ~10% in the UK.
    - M:F = 1:3.

7.9.1 CLINICAL FEATURES

- Based on the Rome II diagnostic criteria:
    - Abdominal discomfort for 12 weeks in the last 12 months with two of these three features:
        - Relieved with defecation.
        - Associated with change in stool frequency.
            - May be increased or decreased.
        - Associated with change in stool form.
            - May be loose or hard.

- Associated symptoms include:
  - Bloating and abdominal distension.
  - Abnormal stool passage:
    - Straining.
    - Urgency.
- Many patients find that attacks may be exacerbated by stress.

7.9.2 DIAGNOSIS

- There are no diagnostic tests for IBS.
- IBS is a diagnosis of exclusion.
  - This means that other causes of the patient's symptoms should be sought, and ruled out, before a diagnosis of IBS is given.
- The following tests should be considered in all patients with IBS-like symptoms:
  - stool culture;
  - coeliac screen;
  - colonoscopy (particularly in patients over 50);
  - blood tests:
    - FBC to rule out anaemia;
    - inflammatory markers;
    - LFTs;
    - TSH to screen for thyroid dysfunction
  - USS.

7.9.3 MANAGEMENT

- Reassurance that there is no underlying, organic pathology.

Lifestyle advice

- Patients should be encouraged to eat a balanced, high-fibre diet.
- Regular exercise and relaxation techniques may help some patients, especially if their symptoms are stress-related.

Laxatives

- Bulking agents (e.g. fybogel) and stool softeners (e.g. lactulose) are indicated in constipation-predominant IBS.

Anti-diarrhoeals

- Opioids (e.g. codeine) or loperamide can be used for symptom relief in diarrhoea-predominant IBS.

Anti-spasmodics

- Medications, such as mebeverine or hyoscine butylbromide, may help with abdominal cramps in a minority of patients.

General surgery

7.10 COLORECTAL CANCER

7.10.1 EPIDEMIOLOGY

- Colorectal cancer is the third most common cancer diagnosis in the UK.
  - It is the second commonest cause of cancer death.
- M:F ratio = M > F.
- It rarely occurs in the under 50s, and is commonest in the over 60s.

7.10.2 AETIOLOGY

- The exact cause is unknown, but there are thought to be several aetiological factors (see Table 7.3).

Table 7.3 Aetiological factors associated with colorectal cancer.

INCREASED RISK	DECREASED RISK
Diet low in fibre.	Exercise.
High-fat and meat diet.	Diet rich in fruit and vegetables.
Inflammatory bowel disease.	Aspirin and non-steroidal anti-inflammatory drug (NSAID) use.
Familial syndromes.	? HRT.
Family history (1 first-degree relative—1:17 risk).	
Poor glycaemic control in diabetics.	

7.10.3 PATHOLOGY

- Histopathologically 98% are adenocarcinomas with characteristic 'signet ring cells' (mucin within the cell).
- They may be well, moderately or poorly differentiated.
- Macroscopically may be papilliferous, polypoid, ulcerated, annular or diffuse.
- Tumours initially invade the lumen, but extend through the bowel wall layers, and eventually through the serosa.
  - The tumour may then spread locally to adjacent organs.
- Lymphatic spread is to the mesenteric and para-aortic nodes.
- Haematogenous spread is to the liver and lungs.
  - Metastases to other sites is uncommon.

- As many as 25% of patients with colorectal cancer have distant metastases at presentation.

> **MICRO-reference**
> Screening for colorectal cancer using the faecal occult blood test: an update. *Cochrane Database of Systematic Reviews* 2006.

7.10.4 CLINICAL FEATURES

- Patients may be symptomatic (see Figure 7.12) or present through the colorectal cancer screening program (faecal occult blood testing).
- Clinical presentations will vary according to the site of the tumour (see Figure 7.13).

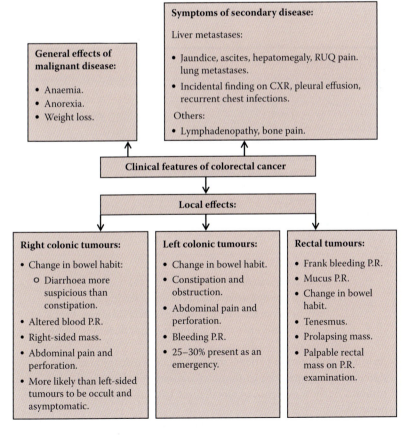

Figure 7.12 Clinical features of colorectal cancer.

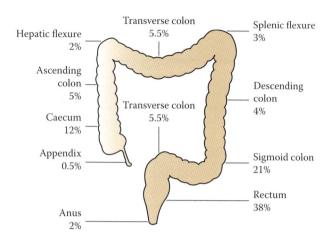

Figure 7.13 Distribution of colorectal cancer. (From: *Bailey & Love's Short Practice of Surgery, 26th Edition*, Figure 69.23, p. 1165.)

MICRO-facts

NHS Bowel Cancer Screening Programme:
- Began in July 2006 with a phased rollout over 3 years across the UK.
- Offers screening every 2 years to all men and women aged 60–69 years.
  - People over 70 can request screening.
- Reduces the risk of dying from bowel cancer by 16%.
- Test is by a home faecal occult blood (FOB) test.
  - If positive patients are called to undergo colonoscopic assessment.

7.10.5 DIAGNOSIS

- Blood tests of use are:
  - FBC (may show anaemia);
  - U&E (useful pre-operatively or in the acute setting);
  - LFT (may be deranged in the presence of liver metastases);
  - Carcinoembryonic antigen (CEA) should be taken as a baseline after confirmation of the diagnosis.
- At initial consultation patients should have proctoscopy and rigid sigmoidoscopy (may allow tumour visualisation in low rectal tumours or show evidence of blood/slime from above; however usually normal).
- Colonoscopy allows visualisation of the entire colon and biopsy.
- Barium enema may show the typical 'apple core' lesion of CRC (Figure 7.14).

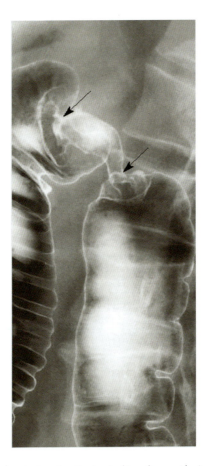

Figure 7.14 Barium enema showing the typical 'apple core' lesion of a colonic carcinoma. (From: *Illustrated Clinical Anatomy, 2nd Edition*, Figure 6.10, p. 94.)

- A negative barium study cannot exclude a small tumour.
- Biopsies are required to give the definitive cellular diagnosis.

7.10.6 STAGING

- Commonly classified according to the modified Duke's criteria (see Table 7.4).
- Most commonly performed with CT scanning.
  - Ultrasound or magnetic resonance imaging (MRI) may better show small liver metastases and chest x-ray may be used to show lung metastases.
  - MRI or trans-rectal USS is used to assess pelvic extent and lymph node status in rectal cancers.

General surgery

Table 7.4 Table showing staging systems and survival of CRC.

TNM CLASSIFICATION		MODIFIED DUKE'S CRITERIA	5-YEAR SURVIVAL
Stage I (N0, M0)	Tumours invade submucosa [T1].	A	85–95%
	Tumours invade muscularis propria [T2].		
Stage IIA (N0, M0)	Tumours invade subserosa [T3].	B	60–80%
Stage IIB	Tumour invades into adjacent organs [T4].		
Stage III (M0)	1–3 regional lymph nodes involved (T1+2) [N1].	C	30–60%
Stage IIIB	1–3 regional lymph nodes involved (T3+4) [N1].		
Stage IIIC	4 or more regional lymph nodes involved [N2].		
Stage IV	Distant metastases [M1].	D	<10%

- PET scanning may also be used to look for extra-hepatic metastases.

7.10.7 TREATMENT

Surgery

- 80% of colorectal cancers will be amenable to resection.
  - May be performed via laparotomy or laparoscopy.
  - The resection is based on the mesenteric blood vessels.
  - Bowel resection with lymphadenectomy is the only curative procedure.
    - For the types of resection, see Figure 7.15.
- For unresectable tumours palliative procedures to prevent obstruction include:
  - endoluminal stents;
  - defunctioning stoma;
  - surgical bypass;
  - debulking palliative resection.
- Some hepatic and, to a lesser extent, pulmonary metastases may be resectable.

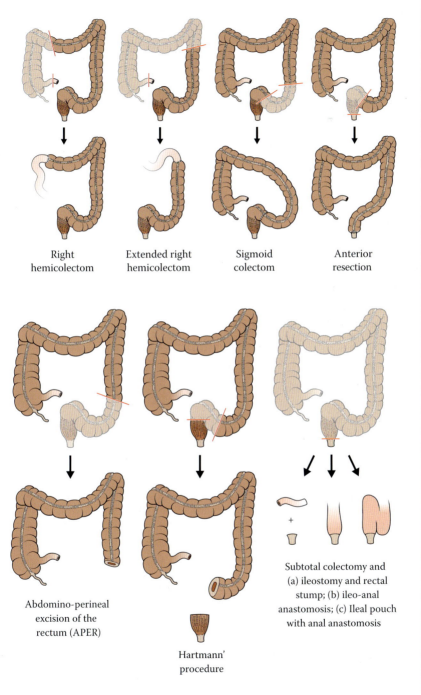

Right hemicolectom

Extended right hemicolectom

Sigmoid colectom

Anterior resection

Abdomino-perineal excision of the rectum (APER)

Hartmann' procedure

Subtotal colectomy and (a) ileostomy and rectal stump; (b) ileo-anal anastomosis; (c) Ileal pouch with anal anastomosis

Figure 7.15 Different colonic resections.

Chemotherapy

- Used in palliation of inoperable disease.
- Used as a neoadjuvant agent to downstage liver metastases prior to surgery.
- Used post-operatively (adjuvant) in patients with Duke's C disease.
  - It is not recommended in Duke's A cancer, but the benefit in Duke's B is still unclear, and so it may be used if there are poor prognostic indicators.
- Most regimes involve folinic acid and IV fluorouracil (or capecitabine, which is the oral prodrug of fluorouracil) plus another agent (e.g. oxaliplatin, irinotecan and cetuximab).

Radiotherapy

- May be given pre-operatively to downstage a rectal tumour, making it easier to remove with clear margins.
- It also reduces local recurrence rates.
  - In smaller, node positive tumours, 'short course' radiotherapy is given every day, lasting for 5 days.
  - In larger, bulky tumours that are invading the circumferential resection margin (CRM), 'long course' radiotherapy is given 5 days a week, lasting for up to 6 weeks.
    - Long-course radiotherapy is usually given in combination with chemotherapy.
    - Fluorouracil (5FU) helps sensitise cells to the effect of radiotherapy.
- Post-operatively, radiotherapy is used in patients who are judged to be at high risk of local recurrence following final histological examination:
  - If the tumour was large and difficult to remove.
  - If the resection margin was not clear.
  - If the tumour had invaded through the bowel wall or there was lymph node involvement.
- It is not used in colon cancer due to the variable positions and risk of small bowel injury.

7.10.8 PROGNOSIS

- Survival depends on the stage of tumour (see Table 7.4).
- Follow-up should be offered to all patients and patients undergoing curative resection should be offered:
  - A minimum of two CT chest, abdomen, pelvis in the first 3 years.
  - Regular CEA tests (6 monthly for 3 years).
  - Surveillance colonoscopy should be offered at 1 year and then again at 5 years.
- Follow-up should be stopped when the risk of investigation outweighs the benefits (length of follow-up is often determined by local cancer networks).

> **MICRO-reference**
> NICE guideline CG131: Colorectal cancer—The diagnosis and management of colorectal cancer.

> **MICRO-case**
> A 65-year-old man presents to his GP with 'problems with haemorrhoids'. He describes blood in his stool and on the toilet paper. However, on further questioning, he has noticed a change in his bowel habit, fluctuating between diarrhoea and constipation. He states that 'his appetite is not what it used to be' and he may have lost some weight.
> Rectal examination reveals a hard mass at the fingertip, and there is some blood and mucus on the glove. Rigid sigmoidoscopy visualises the lesion at around 7 cm. A full colonoscopy is performed to rule out synchronous tumours and for biopsy. Histology confirms adenocarcinoma, and he undergoes further staging investigation for rectal carcinoma.
> **Learning points:**
> - Rectal bleeding in older patients should be investigated for carcinoma of the bowel before a benign diagnosis is given.
> - Many rectal cancers can be palpated on PR examination: 'If you don't put your finger in it, you put your foot in it!'

7.11 COLONIC POLYPS

7.11.1 DEFINITION

- A morphological description of any growth from the wall of the bowel into the lumen.
  - They may be described as sessile (spread over the surface of wall) or pedunculated (hanging from a stalk into the lumen).
- They are usually asymptomatic, but with increasing size or proximity to the anus may cause symptoms such as bleeding or mucous per rectum and prolapse into the anus.
- Polyps may be classified as hamartomas (e.g., juvenile polyps, Peutz-Jeghers syndrome), neoplastic (adenomas) or lymphoid (seen in ulcerative colitis).

7.11.2 FAMILIAL SYNDROMES

Familial adenomatous polyposis

- Arises due to an autosomal dominant defect in the APC gene on chromosome 5.
- There is growth of hundreds to thousands of adenomatous polyps in the colon, which have malignant potential (Figure 7.16).

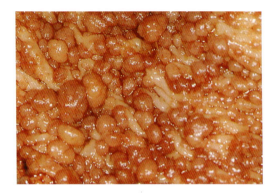

Figure 7.16 Familial adenomatous polyposis. (From: *Bailey & Love's Short Practice of Surgery, 26th Edition*, Figure 65.37, p. 1178.)

- These are on average seen from the age of 16.
- Tracing and screening of families is essential, and affected individuals should be offered prophylactic colectomy.

Hereditary non-polyposis colorectal cancer

- Arises from mutations in the mismatch repair genes (involved in mending the DNA), which causes multiple genetic defects to occur.
- In HNPCC patients develop low numbers of adenomatous polyps that progress more rapidly than normal to cancer.
- There are criteria for HNPCC to be suspected:
  - The modified Amsterdam or Bethesda criteria.

MICRO-facts

Modified Amsterdam criteria:
- Three or more cases of CRC in a minimum of two generations.
- One affected individual must be a first-degree relative.
- One case must be diagnosed at <50 years of age.
- FAP should be excluded.
- Tumours must have pathological verification.

7.11.3 ADENOMA-CARCINOMA SEQUENCE

- This is the sequence from normal tissue to the formation of adenomatous polyps and malignant change.
- It involves multiple genetic changes, and is well demonstrated in the FAP sequence:
  - Inactivation of the APC gene results in bowel epithelial hyperplasia, leading to adenoma formation.

- Activation of oncogenes (e.g. K-ras) increases cellularity, leading to further growth.
- Finally, inactivation of tumour suppressor genes (e.g. p53) leads to carcinoma formation, with uncontrolled tumour growth and angiogenesis.

7.11.4 TREATMENT OF POLYPS

- Polyps need to be removed because of the malignant potential they have.
  - This may be during either colonoscopy:
    - snare excision;
    - endoscopic mucosal resection (EMR).
  - Larger polyps may require operative resection.

7.12 DIVERTICULAR DISEASE

7.12.1 DEFINITION

- A colonic diverticulum is an acquired out-pouching of the mucosa through the circular muscle in the bowel wall (Figure 7.17).

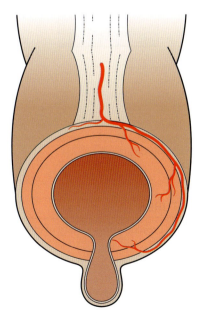

Figure 7.17 Transverse section of the colon with diverticula showing the relationship to the penetrating blood vessels. (From: *Ellis, Lecture Notes*, Figure 25.1, p. 205.)

General surgery

7.12.2 EPIDEMIOLOGY

- More common with increasing age:
  - 10% of people over 40 years; 60% of people over 80.
- Common in the West where a low-fibre diet is prevalent.

7.12.3 PATHOLOGY

- Figure 7.18 describes the process by which colonic diverticula may form.
- Sites of colonic diverticula:
  - 45% sigmoid colon only;
  - 35% sigmoid and descending colon;
  - 10% sigmoid, descending and transverse colon;
  - 5% pancolonic;
  - 5% caecum.

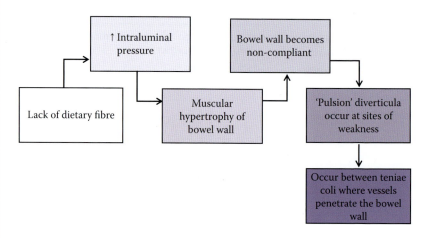

Figure 7.18 Formation of colonic diverticula.

7.12.4 CLINICAL FEATURES

- Diverticular disease may present with a variety of clinical pictures.

7.12.5 DIVERTICULOSIS

- Usually found incidentally at colonoscopy or barium enema.
- May cause vague gastrointestinal symptoms:
  - change in bowel habit (pellet-like stools);
  - bloating and discomfort.
- May be asymptomatic.

7.12.6 DIVERTICULITIS

- Inflammation of the diverticular segment.
- Clinical features:
  - left iliac fossa pain, usually with localised peritonism;
  - systemic features of infection with pyrexia and tachycardia.
- Delayed outpatient investigation should be performed after initial inflammation has settled.

7.12.7 DIVERTICULAR ABSCESS

- Partial localisation of a diverticular perforation.
  - May involve the mesentery, pelvis or retroperitoneum.
- Clinical features:
  - palpable, tender mass in the left iliac fossa with localised peritonism;
  - systemic sepsis with tachycardia, hypotension and spiking pyrexia.

7.12.8 PERITONITIS

- Due to a ruptured abscess or a free perforation.
- Clinical features:
  - presents with an acute abdomen with rigidity and absent bowel sounds;
  - systemic sepsis with shock.

7.12.9 DIVERTICULAR BLEED

- Usually occurs in the absence of inflammation.
- Caused by the erosion of a mural blood vessel by a diverticulum.
- Clinical features:
  - dark red rectal bleeding;
  - may cause an acute drop in haemoglobin.

7.12.10 FISTULAE

- These usually result from recurrent attacks of diverticulitis.
- Usually occur between the sigmoid colon and:
  - Bladder (colovesical fistula).
    - Symptoms include:
      - ○ pneumaturia (passing air in the urine);
      - ○ recurrent urinary tract infections;
      - ○ passage of frank faeces through the urethra.
  - Uterus or vagina.
    - Symptoms include:
      - ○ faecal vaginal discharge with resulting perineal soreness.
  - Skin (colocutaneous).
    - these are very rare.

General surgery

7.12.11 DIVERTICULAR STRICTURE

- Stenosis following fibrotic healing after an episode of diverticulitis.
  - May present with obstructive symptoms.

> ### MICRO-facts
>
> Diverticular vs. malignant strictures:
> - Smooth-walled.
> - No mucosal disruption.
> - No 'apple core' appearance.
> - Tend to be longer.

7.12.12 DIAGNOSIS

- FBC:
  - ↓ Hb in diverticular bleed.
  - ↑ WCC in diverticulitis, abscess or perforation.
- Erect CXR if free perforation is suspected.
- Abdominal x-ray (AXR) if obstruction is suspected.
- CT scan is useful in acute presentations to differentiate between simple diverticulitis and diverticular abscesses or perforations.
- Double-contrast barium enema is useful to demonstrate simple diverticular disease, diverticular strictures or fistulae.
  - Should not be used if perforation or obstruction is suspected due to the risk of causing or exacerbating perforation.
- Colonoscopy is useful in the absence of acute inflammation.
  - Biopsy of strictures may be taken to rule out malignancies.

7.12.13 MANAGEMENT

- Simple measures to improve symptoms of chronic diverticular disease:
  - Increase dietary fibre (e.g. whole-meal bread, rice, fruits, vegetables, bran).
  - Bulking agents (e.g. fybogel).
  - Stool softeners (e.g. lactulose).
  - Anti-spasmodics (e.g. mebeverine).

Acute presentations

- Supportive management:
  - nil by mouth;
  - IV fluid resuscitation;
  - IV antibiotics (e.g. cefuroxime and metronidazole) if septic;
  - blood transfusion if bleeding with symptomatic or severe anaemia;
  - regular observations and reassessment.

General surgery

- Drainage of localised abscess formation:
  - Radiological drainage is successful in ~75% of cases.
- Arrest bleeding:
  - Radiological embolisation or colonoscopic haemostasis.
- Surgery:
  - Emergency laparotomy:
    - Hartmann's procedure (in infective conditions).
    - Sigmoid colectomy.
    - 20% of patients with acute diverticulitis undergo laparotomy for faecal peritonitis, abscesses that are not amenable to radiological drainage, obstruction or bleeding.
  - Emergency laparoscopy may be used for perforation with minimal contamination, allowing washout and placement of drains.
  - Planned resection:
    - For chronic complications (e.g. fistulae).
    - If cancer cannot be excluded.

7.13 ANGIODYSPLASIA

7.13.1 AETIOLOGY

- Small, submucosal vascular anomalies of unknown aetiology.
- Occur in the elderly and so are thought to be degenerative in origin.
- Associations:
  - Hereditary telangiectasia of skin and mouth (Osler–Weber–Rendu syndrome).
  - Aortic valve disease.

7.13.2 CLINICAL FEATURES

- May present with:
  - anaemia;
  - positive Faecal Occult Blood (FOB) test;
  - recurrent small bleeds;
  - acute torrential bleed.
- More common in the right colon.

7.13.3 DIAGNOSIS

- Colonoscopy: Spider naevi-like lesion (Figure 7.19).
- Selective mesenteric angiography: 'Blush' lesion.
  - Must be performed during active bleeding phase.

7.13.4 TREATMENT

- Transfusion in patients with significant or symptomatic anaemia.
- Coagulation at colonoscopy may be curative for small lesions.

General surgery

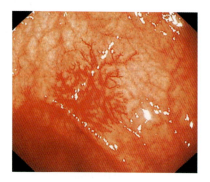

Figure 7.19 Angiodysplasia of the colon as seen on endoscopy. (From: *Bailey & Love's Short Practice of Surgery, 26th Edition*, Figure 11.16, p. 165.)

- Mesenteric embolisation if lesion is visible on angiography.
- Colonic resection (e.g. right hemicolectomy) may be necessary.

7.14 ENDOSCOPY

- Examination via an instrument.
  - Instruments may be rigid or flexible.
- Examples include:
  - Gastroscopy (OGD), colonoscopy, sigmoidoscopy, laparoscopy.
- Benefits and disadvantages are shown in Figure 7.20.

Benefits of Endoscopy:	Disadvantages of Endoscopy:
• Well tolerated. • No general anaesthetic required. • Direct visualisation. • Tissue diagnosis. • More accurate than radiology.	• Small biopsy size. • Specialist training needed. • Specially equipped unit required. • Procedural complications (see below, 7.14.3).

Figure 7.20 Advantages and disadvantages of endoscopy.

7.14.1 PRINCIPLES OF FLEXIBLE ENDOSCOPY

- Flexible fibreoptic fibres transmit light from a high-intensity source in one direction and the image from the lens in the other direction.
- Uses a microchip to transmit the image electronically to a monitor.
- Requires the organs to be inflated (e.g. stomach, bowel) or fluid-filled (bladder).
- Often have a working channel through which instruments can be passed (e.g. biopsy forceps).

- Controlled by rotating levers that manipulate the tip of the endoscope. 'Torque' is applied to the entire endoscope to provide additional rotation.
- Most have end-viewing lenses but some (e.g. the duodenoscope used in endoscopic retrograde cholangiopancreatography (ERCP)) are side-viewing.

7.14.2 USES

Mucosal visualisation
- Diagnosis.
- Screening.
- Follow-up, e.g. following colorectal cancer resection or polypectomy.

CLO test
Histological diagnosis
- Biopsy of lesions.
- Polypectomy.

Therapeutic
- Treatment of bleeding lesions.
    - Adrenaline injection, laser, diathermy.
- Sclerosant injection or banding of oesophageal varices.
- Strictures:
    - Balloon dilatation.
    - Placement of stents.
- Removal of foreign bodies.
- ERCP.
    - Cannulation of ampulla to allow retrograde injection of contrast.
    - Sphincerotomy (ampulla of Vater).
- Percutaneous endoscopic gastrostomy (PEG) insertion.
- Percutaneous endoscopic colostomy (PEC) creation.

7.14.3 COMPLICATIONS

- Perforation:
    - Colonoscopy: <0.5% of diagnostic and <1% of therapeutic procedures.
    - OGD: <1 in 100 000.
- Bleeding (<1%).
- Respiratory depression (when sedation is used).
- Aspiration with gastroscopy.
- Transfer of infection (theoretical risk requiring rigorous sterilisation procedures).
- Cardiovascular complications.
- Mortality (0.01–0.025%).

7.14.4 PATIENT PREPARATION

- Preparation for endoscopy may be divided into general and procedure-specific considerations (see Figure 7.21).

Colonoscopy-specific:

- 7 days before: stop iron.
- 48 hours before: clear liquid diet.
- 12 hours before: laxative preparation.

OGD-specific:

- Fasted overnight prior to procedure.
- Local anaesthetic throat spray.
- Teeth guard.

General Patient Preparation:

- 7 days before: stop anticoagulants (e.g. warfarin, anti-platelets) and consider the need for alternative (such as S.C. low-molecular weight heparin).
- Review for risk factors: coagulopathies, cardiovascular comorbidities, prosthetic heart valves, drug allergies.
- Obtain written informed consent.
- Ensure I.V. access, administer oxygen, monitor vital signs (including oxygen saturation).

Figure 7.21 Patient preparation for endoscopic procedures.

7.15 PILONIDAL DISEASE

7.15.1 DEFINITION

- From the Latin meaning 'nest of hair'.
- Accumulation of hair in pits (usually in natal cleft) leading to infection and abscess formation.

7.15.2 EPIDEMIOLOGY

- M:F = 4:1.
- Occurs in young adulthood, rare after the age of 40 years.
- Typically seen in dark-haired hirsute men.

7.15.3 AETIOLOGY

- Hair from head, back or buttocks is 'driven' into sinus via rolling force from buttock movement with subsequent granulation tissue formation.
- May be multiple.
- Precipitated by sitting and is therefore more common in, e.g. lorry drivers.
- More common in occupations working with hair, e.g. hairdressers and farmers where pilonidal sinuses may occur between fingers.

7.15.4 CLINICAL FEATURES

- Chronic, intermittent purulent discharge from sinus.
- Signs of abscess formation:
    - swelling;
    - erythema;
    - tenderness;
    - fistula formation.

MICRO-facts

It is important to check glucose tolerance in these patients, as recurrent infection may be a presenting feature of diabetes mellitus.

7.15.5 MANAGEMENT

General measures

- Good hygiene, e.g. washing of area.
- Regular depilation, e.g. shaving or waxing of area.

Acute abscess

- Surgical incision and drainage.
    - The incision should be placed off the midline to one side.
- May need antibiotics.

Chronic sinus

- Excision of sinus network and granulation tissue.
- Wound is either left open to heal by secondary intent or closed, usually involving the use of flaps.

Prognosis

- Pilonidal sinus disease usually follows a chronic course with acute exacerbations.
- Recurrence rate is high after surgery.
- Attention to personal hygiene reduces risk of recurrence.

7.16 HAEMORRHOIDS (COMMONLY REFERRED TO AS 'PILES')

7.16.1 DEFINITION

- Congestion of vascular plexuses in anal cushion.

General surgery

> ## MICRO-facts
>
> Classification:
> - **Internal** = of the upper anal canal (i.e. columnar epithelium).
> - **External** = of the lower anal canal (i.e. stratified squamous epithelium).
> - **Grade I** = confined to anal canal.
> - **Grade II** = prolapse of haemorrhoid on defecation with spontaneous reduction.
> - **Grade III** = prolapse during defecation without spontaneous reduction (can reduce digitally).
> - **Grade IV** = permanently prolapsed (cannot be reduced).

7.16.2 EPIDEMIOLOGY

- ~50% of people will suffer from haemorrhoids at some point.
- Tend to occur in young adulthood.
- Men tend to suffer for longer than women.
- More common in Western civilisation due to lack of dietary fibre.

7.16.3 AETIOLOGY

- Anything that increases intra-abdominal pressure will lead to venous engorgement:
  - chronic constipation;
  - straining during defecation;
  - pregnancy.

7.16.4 CLINICAL FEATURES

- More common with increasing age—clinical features are shown in Figure 7.22.

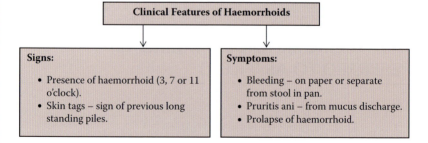

Figure 7.22 Clinical features of haemorrhoids.

7.16.5 INVESTIGATION

- Proctoscopy—to visualise internal haemorrhoids.
- Rigid sigmoidoscopy—to rule out other pathology, e.g. colorectal cancer.
- Colonoscopy—as for rigid sigmoidoscopy.

7.16.6 MANAGEMENT

General measures

- Avoid constipation, i.e. increase dietary fibre, use of laxative.

Banding

- Also known as Barron's banding.
- Placement of rubber bands around the haemorrhoid (if large grade I or grade II) leads to strangulation, thrombosis and subsequent dropping off of the haemorrhoid.
- Performed during proctoscopy.

Sclerotherapy

- Proctoscopic injection of 1–3 mL of 5% phenol in almond oil above each haemorrhoid.
    - Cannot be used in patients who have a nut allergy.
- Promotes thrombosis of haemorrhoid.
- May need repeating.

Operative interventions

- Reserved for grade III haemorrhoids.
- Open haemorrhoidectomy:
    - Excision of haemorrhoid plus overlying mucosa and skin with arterial ligation.
    - Important to leave skin bridges between resection areas; otherwise anal stenosis may occur.
- Stapled haemorrhoidopexy.
    - Uses a surgical staple gun to circumferentially excise a ring of haemorrhoidal tissue, leaving a stapled anastomosis.

7.16.7 COMPLICATIONS

Thrombosis/strangulated pile

- Presents with acute pain.
- Usually resolves spontaneously; therefore give analgesic and cold compress.
- May need haemorrhoidectomy.

General surgery

7.17 RECTAL PROLAPSE

7.17.1 DEFINITION

- Herniation of variable layers of rectal wall through the pelvic floor.
- Can be partial thickness (rectal mucosa only) or full thickness (all layers of rectal wall).

7.17.2 EPIDEMIOLOGY

- Occurs in young children (partial thickness) and elderly women (full thickness).

7.17.3 AETIOLOGY

- Straining during defecation.
- Constipation.
- Multiple vaginal deliveries.
- Poor sphincter tone.
- Rarely, they may be caused by a cancer as the lead point.

7.17.4 CLINICAL FEATURES

- Presence of prolapse.
- Incontinence (full-thickness prolapse) due to dilatation of anal sphincter leading to decreased tone.
- Mucus discharge.
- Pruritis ani.
- Incomplete defecation.
- Rectal bleeding.

7.17.5 MANAGEMENT

- Avoidance of straining and constipation.
- Usually resolves spontaneously in children and parental reassurance is all that is necessary.
- Sclerotherapy can be effective in partial-thickness prolapse.
- Surgical management:
    - Delorme's perianal rectopexy:
        - Per-anal excision of excess mucosa with plication of rectum to prevent subsequent prolapse.
    - Altmier's rectosigmoidectomy:
        - Perineal excision of the affected excess rectosigmoid with anastomosis.
    - Transabdominal rectopexy:
        - With or without resection of part of the sigmoid colon.
        - Rectal mobilisation and fixation with sutures to the presacral fascia.

 – Higher success rate than perianal approach, although less suitable for frail elderly women.
 – May be performed laparoscopically.

7.18 ANAL FISSURE

7.18.1 DEFINITION

- Longitudinal tear in anal mucosa.
- 90% occur in the posterior midline of anal mucosa.

7.18.2 EPIDEMIOLOGY

- M:F ratio M = F.
- More common in young adults.

7.18.3 AETIOLOGY

- Constipation and passage of hard stools (see Figure 7.23).

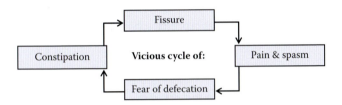

Figure 7.23 Aetiological cycle of anal fissure.

- Can occur after anal intercourse or vigorous wiping.
- Associated with Crohn's and UC, where they may be multiple.
- Anterior fissures are associated with obstetric trauma.

7.18.4 CLINICAL FEATURES

- Acute pain on defecation—'knife-like'.
- History of constipation.
- Bright red blood on paper.
- Pain on anal wiping.
- May be presence of skin tag at superficial end of fissure (sentinel pile).
- Excess pain on PR examination; therefore should not be performed.

7.18.5 MANAGEMENT

Medical

- Avoidance of constipation, e.g. use of laxatives.
- Glyceryl tri-nitrate (GTN) ointment 0.2–0.4% to relax anal sphincter and dilate vessels, thus promoting healing.

General surgery

- Diltiazem ointment may be effective if GTN fails.

Botox therapy

- Local injection of botulinum A injection aims to break the spasm-fissure cycle.
- Usually injected under general anaesthetic in theatre.

Surgical

- Lateral internal sphincterotomy:
  - Division of internal sphincter.
  - Risk of incontinence, especially if past medical history of obstetric trauma.
- Anal advancement flap:
  - Excision of the fissure that is covered with a piece of mucosa that is rotated as a flap from above.

MICRO-print

Lord's anal stretch:

- Dilatation (under anaesthetic) of anal sphincter using <4 fingers.
- Unacceptably high rates of incontinence and should no longer be used.

7.19 ANORECTAL ABSCESS

7.19.1 AETIOLOGY

- Acute infection of anal glands with subsequent spread to adjacent perianal structures (see Figure 7.24).
- If presence of concurrent fistula-in-ano, abscesses are likely to be recurrent.

7.19.2 CLINICAL FEATURES

- Localised perianal pain.

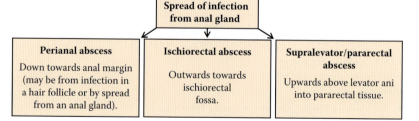

Spread of infection from anal gland		
Perianal abscess	**Ischiorectal abscess**	**Supralevator/pararectal abscess**
Down towards anal margin (may be from infection in a hair follicle or by spread from an anal gland).	Outwards towards ischiorectal fossa.	Upwards above levator ani into pararectal tissue.

Figure 7.24 Classification and aetiology of anorectal abscesses.

- Erythema.
- Swelling (perianal abscess).
- If supralevator or ischiorectal abscess there may be no superficial signs, but tenderness on abdominal examination is common.
- Systemic signs of infection, e.g. fever, rigors and tachycardia.

7.19.3 MANAGEMENT

- If early, oral antibiotics may settle the infection.
- Surgical incision and drainage is the definitive treatment.
- Important to send a swab of pus to differentiate the origin of the bacterium, i.e. colonic (may indicate fistula) or skin organism.

7.20 FISTULA-IN-ANO

7.20.1 DEFINITION

- Abnormal communication between two epithelialised surfaces—in this case between the anal mucosa and the perineal/vaginal skin.

7.20.2 EPIDEMIOLOGY

- Common.
- Occurs in young adulthood.

7.20.3 AETIOLOGY

- Usually from anorectal abscess (may result following surgical drainage).
- Associated with:
    - inflammatory bowel disease, most commonly Crohn's disease;
    - rectal carcinoma;
    - tuberculosis and HIV (both rare).

7.20.4 CLASSIFICATION

- Fistulae are named in relation to the external sphincter; however treatment is decided based on how much internal sphincter is involved (see Figure 7.25).

MICRO-print

Goodsall's rule:

- For prediction of site of the internal opening of low anal fistula.
- The anus is divided transversely (imaginary line).
- **External opening anterior to line:** Short course of fistula into anal canal.
- **External opening posterior to line:** Longer curved course of fistula opening into the anus at the posterior midline.

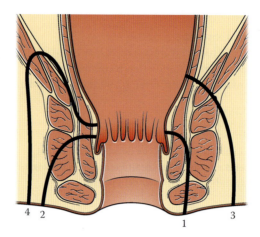

Figure 7.25 Parks' classification of anal fistulae. Type 1: Intersphincteric. Type 2: Trans-sphincteric. Type 3: Suprasphincteric. Type 4: Extrasphincteric. (From: *Bailey & Love's Short Practice of Surgery, 26th Edition,* Figure 73.40, p. 1260.)

7.20.5 CLINICAL FEATURES

- Chronic discharge: Faecally stained mucus/pus.
- Features of anorectal abscess (see Section 7.19).
- External opening on examination.

7.20.6 INVESTIGATION

PR exam

- Can feel the granulation tissue of the fibrosed track.

Examination under anaesthetic (EUA)

- To assess course, as examination while awake will be too painful.
- Insertion of probe into fistula identifies course.

Ultrasound scan or MRI

- Useful to identify course if examination under anaesthetic (EUA) unsuccessful.

7.20.7 MANAGEMENT

Low anal fistula

- Fistulotomy:
  - Division of tissue with scalpel down to the probe inserted during EUA along with excision of granulomatous tissue.
  - Fistula laid open to heal by secondary intent.

– Patient retains continence, as sphincter only minimally/not transected.

High anal fistula

- Seton insertion:
  - Lower part of the fistula is laid open as described above, as complete division of the sphincter would lead to incontinence.
  - A loose seton (thread) is passed through the rest of the fistula, secured and left in place.
    - ◯ This allows drainage of pus and resolution of local sepsis, preventing abscess formation.
    - ◯ Setons allow planning of further definitive treatment.
  - Tight 'cutting' setons can be placed that gradually cut through the muscle over time, allowing healing to occur behind them.

7.21 ANAL CANCER

7.21.1 AETIOLOGY

- Human papilloma virus (HPV) is thought to predispose to anal carcinoma by the process of anal intra-epithelial neoplasia (AIN).

High-risk groups

- Male homosexuals.
- Individuals who practice anal sex.
- Previous history of genital warts.

> **MICRO-print**
> The remaining 20% are comprised of malignant melanomas, lymphomas, Kaposi's sarcoma and anal gland adenocarcinoma.

7.21.2 PATHOLOGY

- 80% are squamous cell carcinomas (SCCs).
- Metastatic spread is commonly to the inguinal lymph nodes.
  - May also spread to the bones and liver.

7.21.3 CLINICAL FEATURES

- Usually presents in the sixth and seventh decade with the following:
  - bleeding from anal canal;
  - perianal pain, swelling and ulceration.
- Late cases may present with:
  - incontinence;

- recto-vaginal fistulae;
- disruption to bowel habit.

7.21.4 DIAGNOSIS

- Examination under anaesthetic (EUA) is performed to assess disease extent and for biopsy confirmation.
- CT scanning may be required to assess for metastatic spread.
- MRI is used for local staging.

7.21.5 TREATMENT

Chemo-radiotherapy

- Usually first-line treatment.
- 4–5 weeks of radiotherapy, including the tumour site and inguinal lymph nodes.
- The chemotherapy regime is usually with IV fluorouracil (5FU) plus mitomicin C or cisplatin.
- Curative in 50%.
- Side effects include:
    - temporary perineal desquamation;
    - induction of artificial menopause in women;
    - azoospermia in males;
    - GI effects, including nausea and diarrhoea;
    - hair loss;
    - neutropenia.

Local surgical resection

- Suitable for small tumours (<2 cm) at the anal margin with no sphincter involvement.
- <5% of patients are suitable for this.

Abdomino-perineal resection (APR)

- Radical major surgery to remove the ano-rectum with a permanent colostomy.
- Reserved for:
    - residual disease following chemo-radiotherapy;
    - disease recurrence.

Diversion colostomy

- May be used to divert the passage of faeces from the perineum during treatment.

7.21.6 PROGNOSIS

- There is a 50% survival rate at 5 years.

7.22 STOMAS

7.22.1 DEFINITION

- The word 'stoma' is Greek for 'mouth'.
- A stoma in surgery is a surgically created opening of the gastrointestinal tract (or urinary tract) onto the abdominal wall.

MICRO-facts

Indications for stomas:
- Feeding (e.g. following CVA).
- Diversion of faeces (away from a distal anastomosis or distal disease.
- Exteriorisation (when primary anastomosis is not possible or following proctectomy).

7.22.2 CLASSIFICATION

- Stomas may be classified by their site, permanence or number of lumens (i.e. end or loop).

Site

- Gastrostomy (stomach, e.g. PEG). They are usually placed in the epigastrium.
- Jejunostomy (jejunum).
- Ileostomy (ileum: small bowel stomas have a spout to protect skin from the alkaline bowel content and active enzymes) (see Figure 7.26a). They produce liquid bowel content and are usually sited in the RIF.
- Ileal conduit (anastomosis of the ureters to one end of a detached segment of ileum following cystectomy, with the other end forming a stoma for urinary drainage).
- Colostomy (colon: these are flush against the skin) (see Figure 7.26b). They usually produce solid faeces and are most commonly sited in the LIF.

Permanence

- Temporary:
    - To protect a distal anastomosis.
    - To defunction distal bowel to allow healing.
    - If primary anastomosis should not be performed, e.g. in the presence of sepsis.
- Permanent:
    - Following proctectomy (e.g. panproctocolectomy, AP resection).
    - If primary anastomosis is not possible for technical reasons.

General surgery

(a)

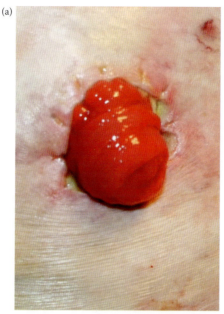

(b)

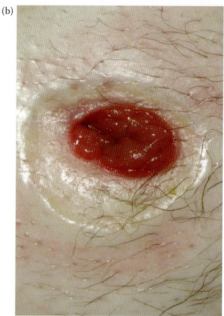

Figure 7.26 (a) End ileostomy – Note the spout to keep the succus entericus from coming in contact with the skin. (b) End colostomy, which is flush with the skin. [From: personal photographs (consent obtained from patients).]

7.22.3 SITING

- A suitable site should be selected and marked pre-operatively by a specialist stoma nurse whenever possible.
    - Assess the abdomen lying and standing for best positioning.
    - Assess clothed, as waistbands may cause problems with stoma devices.
    - Ensure good visibility to enable patients to manage the stoma themselves.

Areas to avoid
- The wound site.
- Existing scars.
- The umbilicus.
- Bony prominences.

7.22.4 COMPLICATIONS

Technical
- Ischaemia, may be due to:
    - Excessive tension on bowel mesentery, causing vessel injury.
    - Tight abdominal wall defect causing compression.
- Prolapse.
- Retraction.
- Parastomal hernia.
    - Risk of bowel obstruction or strangulation within the hernia.
- Stenosis, may be due to:
    - ischaemia;
    - underlying disease process.

General
- High-output:
    - Due to shortened bowel proximal to stoma.
    - Can cause dehydration and electrolyte disturbances.
- Nutritional disorders:
    - Vitamin B deficiency (megaloblastic anaemia).
- Gallstones:
    - In small bowel stomas, as the terminal ileum is bypassed and this is where bile salts are absorbed.

8 Vascular

8.1 VASCULAR ANATOMY

- The major bloods vessels are shown in Figure 8.1.

8.2 AAA

8.2.1 DEFINITION

- Arterial aneurysms are a permanent abnormal dilatation of the vessel to a diameter of 50% or more than that of the non-dilated vessel.
- Regarding the abdominal aorta, this is generally ≥3 cm in AP diameter.

8.2.2 EPIDEMIOLOGY

- M:F ratio = 6:1.
- Incidence increases with age (occurring in 7–8% of men over 65 years).

8.2.3 AETIOLOGY

- Generally caused by atherosclerotic degeneration of the intima and media, leading to weakening of arterial wall.
- Associated with connective tissue disorders, e.g. Marfan's syndrome or Ehlers–Danlos syndrome.
- Secondary to abdominal trauma.
- Infections, e.g. tertiary syphilis, *Salmonella typhi*, *Escherichia coli*.

Risk factors

- Smoking.
- Hypercholesterolaemia.
- Hypertension.
- Family history.

8.2.4 PATHOLOGY

- Commonly occur below the renal arteries.
- May be associated with an aneurysm of the femoral or popliteal arteries in ~25%.
- Usually fusiform in shape but may be saccular (see Figure 8.2).
- May throw off thromboemboli.

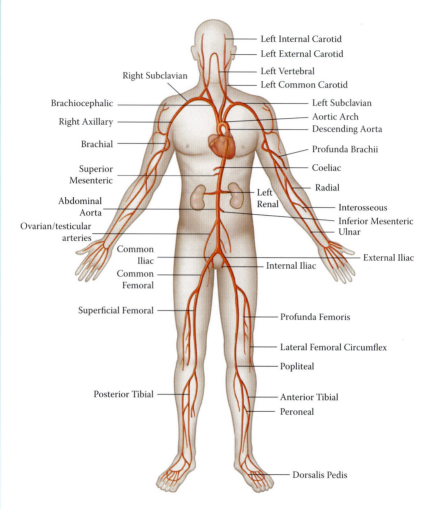

Figure 8.1 The main (a) arteries and (b) veins. (From: authors' own renderings.)

8.2.5 CLINICAL FEATURES

- Usually asymptomatic and found incidentally when investigating other abdominal pathology.
- Symptoms may arise following complications of leakage, rupture or from thromboemboli (Figure 8.3).
- Abdominal and back pain from expansion.
- Pulsatile expansile mass in epigastric/umbilical region.

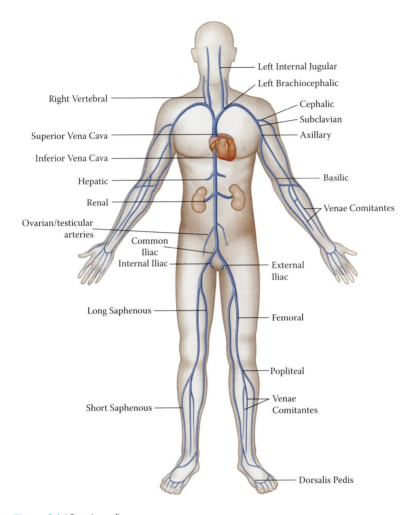

Figure 8.1 (*Continued*)

8.2.6 INVESTIGATIONS

- Ultrasound scan (USS) is the test of choice for assessing size of aneurysm.
- Computer tomography (CT) is good for assessing size and relation to other abdominal structures.
  - Three-dimensional reconstruction can be used to plan surgical intervention.

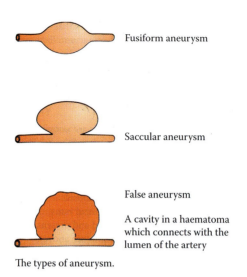

Fusiform aneurysm

Saccular aneurysm

False aneurysm

A cavity in a haematoma which connects with the lumen of the artery

The types of aneurysm.

Figure 8.2 The types of aneurysms. (From: *Browse's Introduction to the Symptoms and Signs of Surgical Disease, 4th Edition*, Figure 7.9, p. 190.)

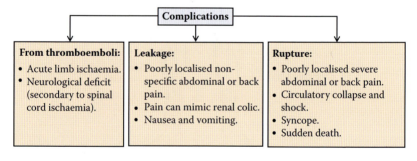

Complications		
From thromboemboli:	**Leakage:**	**Rupture:**
• Acute limb ischaemia. • Neurological deficit (secondary to spinal cord ischaemia).	• Poorly localised non-specific abdominal or back pain. • Pain can mimic renal colic. • Nausea and vomiting.	• Poorly localised severe abdominal or back pain. • Circulatory collapse and shock. • Syncope. • Sudden death.

Figure 8.3 Complications of AAA.

8.2.7 MANAGEMENT

- Medical management of abdominal aortic aneurysm (AAA) < 5.5 cm:
  - cessation of smoking;
  - aggressive control of hypertension;
  - statin to lower cholesterol;
  - anti-platelet therapy;
  - monitor patients with known AAA < 5.5 cm with regular USS.
- Surgical management may be divided into open or endovascular repair (Figure 8.4).

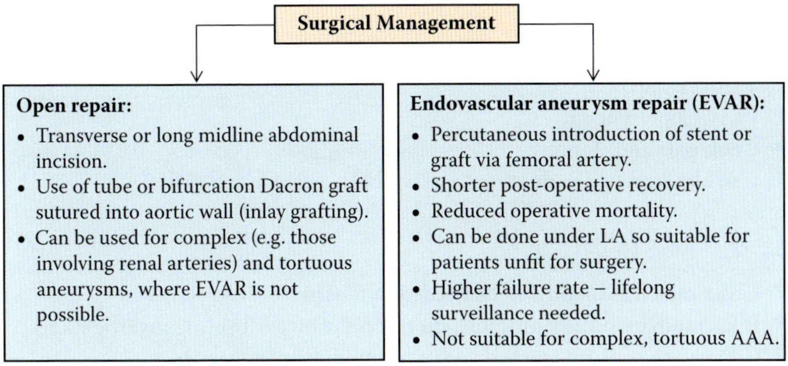

Figure 8.4 Management of AAA.

MICRO-facts

Indications for surgery:
- Diameter ≥ 5.5 cm.
- Diameter increasing by >1 cm per annum.
- Symptomatic aneurysm (may indicate imminent rupture).
- Thromboembolic event secondary to aneurysm.
- Rupture—emergency.

8.2.8 PROGNOSIS

- Rupture rate increases with the following factors:
  - rapid expansion (>1 cm/year) irrespective of size;
  - symptomatic irrespective of size;
  - increase in diameter (<1% per year if < 5.5cm, ~25% if >7 cm).
- Mortality after rupture:
  - 75% die before reaching hospital.
  - The mortality rate remains high even with operative repair in the emergency setting.
- Operative mortality of elective open repair = 5%.

8.3 HOW TO MANAGE A SUSPECTED LEAKING AAA

8.3.1 CLINICAL FEATURES

- Severe non-specific abdominal or back pain.

General surgery

Signs of shock

- Hypotension.
- Tachycardia.
- Presyncope/syncope.
- Cold, pale and clammy.
- Can also lead to disseminated intravascular coagulation (DIC).

8.3.2 INVESTIGATIONS

- Cross-match as blood will be needed in theatre.
- If haemodynamically unstable, **do not** delay by performing investigations.
- CT scan to confirm any leakage (if haemodynamically stable).

8.3.3 MANAGEMENT

ABCDE approach

- Ensure adequate IV access and O_2 therapy is given.
- Call seniors and anaesthetic team early.
- Patients in district general hospitals should be transferred immediately to a tertiary centre with an on-call vascular service.
- Urgent open repair via laparotomy is indicated with inlay grafting (see above).
- Do not aggressively fluid resuscitate as excess fluid can disrupt containment of the rupture within retroperitoneal tissues, leading to exsanguination into the peritoneal cavity.

8.4 AORTIC DISSECTION

8.4.1 DEFINITION

- Tear in the wall of the thoracic aorta leading to splitting of the media.
- Blood forces along a cleavage plane for a variable distance along aorta.

MICRO-facts

Stanford classification (Figure 8.5):
- Type A (most common):
  - Involves the ascending aorta ± the aortic arch.
  - May involve aortic valve leading to regurgitation.
- Type B:
  - Involves descending aorta distal to the left subclavian artery.

8.4.2 EPIDEMIOLOGY

- Incidence = 1 per 100 000 per year.
- Affects men more commonly than women.

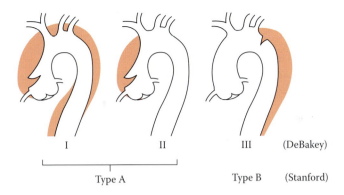

I   II   III   (DeBakey)

Type A   Type B   (Stanford)

Figure 8.5 The Stanford classification of aortic dissection. (From: *Bailey & Love's Short Practice of Surgery, 26th Edition*, Figure 51.28.)

8.4.3 AETIOLOGY

- Hypertension.
- Trauma.
- Connective tissue disorders (e.g. Marfan's or Ehlers–Danlos syndrome).

8.4.4 CLINICAL FEATURES

- See Figure 8.6.
- Presentation may be with sudden death.
  - Type A dissection has a 1% mortality rate per hour from aortic rupture, aortic regurgitation, pericardial tamponade or coronary ischaemia.

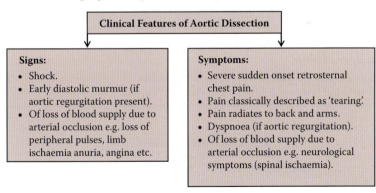

Clinical Features of Aortic Dissection

Signs:
- Shock.
- Early diastolic murmur (if aortic regurgitation present).
- Of loss of blood supply due to arterial occlusion e.g. loss of peripheral pulses, limb ischaemia anuria, angina etc.

Symptoms:
- Severe sudden onset retrosternal chest pain.
- Pain classically described as 'tearing'.
- Pain radiates to back and arms.
- Dyspnoea (if aortic regurgitation).
- Of loss of blood supply due to arterial occlusion e.g. neurological symptoms (spinal ischaemia).

Figure 8.6 Clinical features of aortic dissection.

8.4.5 INVESTIGATIONS

- ECG to exclude MI as cause for chest pain.
- Chest x-ray (CXR) may demonstrate mediastinal widening.
- CT scanning is the gold standard investigation to assess extent of dissection.

General surgery

8.4.6 MANAGEMENT

Type A
- Rapid control of blood pressure.
- Urgent surgical aortic arch replacement is indicated.
  - May need replacement of aortic valve if involved.

Type B
- Principally the management is with medical therapy with aggressive treatment of hypertension.
- If aortic rupture, occlusion of a visceral artery or lower limb ischaemia occurs, urgent surgery is indicated with either open surgery or endovascular treatment.

8.5 ACUTE LIMB ISCHAEMIA

- Acute limb ischaemia (ALI) is a surgical emergency. It requires definite treatment within 6 hours of symptom onset in order to preserve the limb.

8.5.1 EPIDEMIOLOGY
- Incidence of around 14 per 100 000.

8.5.2 AETIOLOGY
- Commonly caused by thrombotic or embolic events (see Figure 8.7).

> ## MICRO-facts
> Thrombotic ALI can be preceded by intermitted claudication, in which case there may be reduced or absent pulses in the contralateral limb.

> ## MICRO-facts
> Aortic dissection often mimics an MI and indeed may precipitate an MI (due to occlusion of coronary arteries).

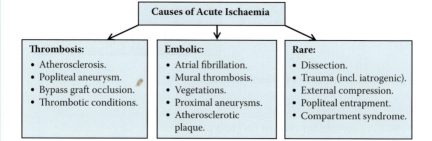

Figure 8.7 Causes of ALI.

8.5.3 CLINICAL PRESENTATION

> **MICRO-facts**
>
> - The classical symptoms of ALI are the 'six P's':
>   - pain;
>   - pallor;
>   - paraesthesia (pins and needles/numbness);
>   - pulseless;
>   - paralysis;
>   - perishing cold.
> - The presence of neurological symptoms (paraesthesia and paralysis— there may be associated muscle tenderness) is a late feature and suggests muscle infarction.

- There may be evidence of embolic source, such as AF or infective endocarditis.
- Other features include:
  - Dehydration, malignancy, inherited clotting disorders (increased thrombosis preponderance).
  - Recent MI with mural thrombosis (source of emboli).
  - A palpable aneurysm (popliteal, abdominal) may be the source of emboli.

8.5.4 INVESTIGATIONS

Blood tests

- Full blood count (FBC), urea and electrolytes (U&E) (the patient may have concomitant renovascular disease), clotting, glucose, cross-match.
- ABG may demonstrate a lactic, metabolic acidosis.
- ECG may reveal AF.
- Doppler scanning to detect blood flow within the limb.
  - Performed at pulse points and can help to determine level of occlusion.
- Arteriography to demonstrate occlusions and assess run-off vessels.
  - This can be performed intra-operatively if an embolic cause is suspected, minimising delay.

8.5.5 DEFINITIVE MANAGEMENT

- For general acute management of ALI please see Section 8.6.
- This is dependent on the underlying cause of the ischaemia:
  - Embolism:
    - Surgical embolectomy, either under local/regional or general anaesthetic.
    - A Fogarty catheter is inserted proximally and distally to the lesion, a balloon inflated and the embolus is removed using the catheter.

- Thrombosis:
  - Thrombolysis is useful in both thrombotic and embolic events. It breaks down clot and prevents further propagation.
  - May be followed by arterial bypass surgery (using autogenous grafts, e.g. long saphenous vein, or synthetic depending on the vessel size involved) or angioplasty.

8.5.6 COMPLICATIONS OF ALI

- Death (20%).
- Limb loss (30%).
  - Irreversible tissue ischaemia may occur within 6 hours.

Reperfusion injury

- Reperfusion of an ischaemic limb results in the reintroduction of blood from that limb into the systemic circulation.
- This blood has a low pH and high potassium concentration and results in a systemic inflammatory response, consequences of which may include multiple organ dysfunction, including renal and pulmonary failure.

Compartment syndrome

- Fluid accumulation within the fascial compartments may occur following revascularisation.
- This raises the intracompartmental pressure to above capillary perfusion pressure, leading to further muscle and nerve damage if not promptly decompressed.

Complications of arterial surgery

- Haemorrhage.
- Thrombosis of grafts leading to distal ischaemia.
- Graft infection.
- Death.

8.6 HOW TO MANAGE A CASE OF POSSIBLE ALI

8.6.1 IMMEDIATE RESUSCITATION

- The patient will be acutely unwell, and so needs emergency resuscitation.
- Give high-flow oxygen to increase oxygen delivery to the affected limb.
- Ensure IV access is available and commence immediate fluid resuscitation.
- Send blood for FBC, U&E, coagulation screen and cross-match.
- Give adequate analgesia, e.g. morphine IV (titrate dose according to patient's age, fitness and level of pain) and adequate anti-emetic cover.

- Call for senior and anaesthetic support early to give the best chance of limb salvage.
  - Immediate transfer to a vascular unit via blue-light ambulance is necessary in hospitals without an on-site vascular service.
- May require anticoagulation with a bolus of 5000 IU of heparin and aspirin.
  - Caution: Patients may be unfit to undergo a general anaesthetic and so anticoagulation should be deferred if regional anaesthesia is required.
  - If the cause is found to be an embolus, then the anticoagulation is converted to oral medication post-operatively.
  - Anticoagulation should always be discussed with senior colleagues before it is commenced.

8.6.2 ESTABLISH THE DIAGNOSIS

Clinical assessment

- Look for the 'six Ps'; remember—paralysis and paraesthesia are late signs.
  - Use both palpation and a handheld Doppler to assess pulses.

Angiography

- Either pre-operative or intra-operative 'on table'.

8.6.3 LIMB VIABILITY ASSESSMENT

- The acutely ischaemic limb can be split into three subgroups: viable, threatened and irreversible, and these influence management.
  - **Viable:** The limb is not immediately threatened and has audible arterial signals on Doppler. This tends to present with the acute onset of rest pain (without paralysis or sensory loss), which is one of the defining symptoms of critical limb ischaemia (the terminal phase of chronic limb ischaemia). As the limb is not in immediate danger, there is time to perform investigations and plan treatment.
  - **Threatened:** The limb viability is threatened and will not survive without urgent treatment. This is the typical 'acute white leg with sensorimotor deficit'.
  - **Irreversible:** The limb is not salvageable. There is fixed mottling with muscle paralysis and tense, swollen fascial compartments. These patients may be treated with primary amputation following adequate resuscitation and stabilisation.

> **MICRO-print**
> Remember: Even though limb ischaemia is most commonly seen in the lower limbs, it can also occur in the upper limbs. The symptoms, signs, investigations and management options remain the same.

General surgery

MICRO-case

A 55-year-old woman presents to the emergency department with excruciating pain in her left leg for the last 2 hours. On examination the leg is cold and white. There is a strong left femoral pulse but no palpable pulses below this, in contrast to the right side where there are strong foot pulses. She is clinically in AF.

She is commenced on high-flow oxygen, IV fluid resuscitation and given morphine and aspirin. She proceeds straight to the operating theatre where she is given IV heparin and an intra-operative angiogram confirms an embolus in the superficial femoral artery. An embolectomy is performed and blood flow is restored to the limb. She is started on warfarin post-operatively.

Learning points:

- Acute limb ischaemia is a clinical diagnosis denoted by acute onset of symptoms with some or all of the 'six P's' being present.
- Patients with embolic events will often present in AF.
- This woman has a threatened leg—this is an emergency and surgery should not be delayed, as there is a 6-hour window between onset of symptoms and irreversible ischaemic damage.

8.7 CHRONIC LOWER LIMB ISCHAEMIA

8.7.1 EPIDEMIOLOGY

- Approximately 15% of the middle-aged and elderly population have evidence of lower limb peripheral arterial disease.
  - Around 5% of these have symptoms.
- The prevalence of critical limb ischaemia is estimated at approximately 1 in 2500 of the population annually.

MICRO-facts

Risk factors:
- Smoking.
- Diabetes.
- Hypercholesterolaemia.
- Hypertension.
- Family history of hyperhomocysteinaemia.

8.7.2 AETIOLOGY

- This is almost entirely due to atherosclerosis and is usually due to smoking.
  - Other rarer causes include:
    - arteritis;
    - Buerger's disease (thromboangiitis obliterans, seen in young male smokers);
    - Takayasu's disease.

8.7.3 CLINICAL PRESENTATION

Intermittent claudication

- This is the main complaint of patients with symptomatic chronic ischaemia.
- It is a severe muscle cramp which occurs on exercise (usually walking), and resolves within minutes of resting.
- Exercise tolerance may worsen over time.
- Symptoms may occur bilaterally.
- Claudication is usually felt in the calf but may occur in the thigh or buttocks depending on the affected vessel.

> **MICRO-print**
> Ensure that reduced exercise tolerance is due to leg pain and that chest pain or shortness of breath is not the limiting factor.

Critical ischaemia

- There may be rest pain, often worse at night, which is a constant pain felt in the affected foot, often improved by hanging the foot over the side of the bed.
- There may be tissue loss with either ischaemic ulceration or gangrene.
- Signs of peripheral vascular disease:
  - These depend on the degree of ischaemia present.
    - There may be reduced or absent pulses on the affected side.
    - In more severe ischaemia, there may be trophic skin changes, e.g. nail thickening, skin atrophy and hairless skin.
    - Buerger's test (see Section 8.8.5) may be positive with more severe degrees of ischaemia.

8.7.4 INVESTIGATIONS

- If there is evidence of other cardiovascular disease, this should be investigated and treated.
  - Patients with chronic limb ischaemia are more likely to die of MI and stroke than of their limb problems.

Bloods

- FBC (thrombocythaemia, polycythaemia, severe anaemia), U&E (renovascular disease), clotting, ESR (arteritis), lipids, glucose (for diabetes), syphilis serology.
- Patients need blood pressure (BP) testing in both arms, and their ankle brachial pressure index (ABPI) calculated.
  - Ankle pressure may be misleadingly high if there is calcification of the vessel (such as in diabetes mellitus), leading to non-compliance.
- Assess the severity of symptoms using a treadmill test.

General surgery

- Duplex Doppler scanning to look for stenosis and occlusion.
- Arteriography and MR angiogram are used in patients in whom angioplasty or reconstructive vascular surgery is being considered.

8.7.5 PROGNOSIS

- There is evidence to suggest that 50% of patients with intermittent claudication will remain stable or demonstrate spontaneous improvement over a 5-year period.
- Approximately 25% of claudicants will have deterioration of their symptoms.
    - 5% of these will require revascularisation.
    - 1–2% will require major amputation.

8.7.6 MANAGEMENT

- Conservative management is often all that is needed.
    - Lifestyle modification:
        - smoking cessation;
        - weight loss;
        - regular exercise;
        - improve diabetic control.
    - Medication:
        - controlling hypertension (though beta-blockers should be avoided);
        - anti-platelet agents;
        - statin.
- If this fails or if the patient has disabling claudication or critical ischaemia, then angioplasty ± stenting or reconstructive arterial surgery may be required (see Figure 8.8).

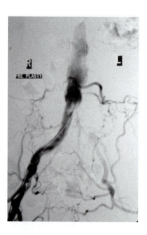

Figure 8.8 Angiogram showing iliac occlusion. (From: *Clinical Surgery: A Practical Guide*, Figure 17.5, p. 239.)

- Surgery carries a significant mortality rate, and is usually reserved for fit patients.
  - There is a significant failure rate. The more distal the vessel, the lower the % graft patency at 2 years (90% in above knee, 50% in distal below knee).
- Ultimately, some patients will undergo major amputation.

> ## MICRO-facts
> Critical ischaemia:
> - Defined by one or more of the following:
>   - Persistent rest pain needing analgesia for >2 weeks.
>   - Ulceration or gangrene.
>   - Ankle systolic pressure of less than 50 mmHg.
> - Can be acute and present as acute limb ischaemia (see Section 8.5) on a background of chronic symptoms.
> - Requires more urgent investigation and treatment to prevent limb loss due to progressive tissue necrosis or infection.

8.8 HOW TO EXAMINE THE PERIPHERAL VASCULAR SYSTEM

8.8.1 GENERAL INSPECTION

- Inspect the surroundings for clues, e.g. glyceryl tri-nitrate (GTN) suggesting IHD, cigarettes, etc.

8.8.2 INSPECTION OF THE PATIENT

General
- Comfort (look for evidence of rest pain).
- Build (ischaemia is associated with obesity, as is diabetes).
- Position (is one leg hung over the edge of the bed or propped on a stool?).

Hands
- Cyanosis.
- Capillary refill.
- Nicotine staining.

Face and eyes
- Corneal arcus (hyperlipidaemia).
- Conjunctival pallor (anaemia).
- Mucous membranes (dehydration).
- Tongue (central cyanosis).

General surgery

Abdomen

- Look for scars, masses, visible pulsations (may indicate AAA).

Legs and feet

- Swelling.
- Colour (red may be a misleading colour due to dependency, e.g. 'sunset foot').
- Trophic changes (loss of hair, shiny skin, venous eczema, ulceration). Remember to check between the toes for ulcers.

8.8.3 PALPATION

Pulses

- Radial: Assess rate and rhythm (is the patient in AF?), and assess radio-radial delay.
- Perform Allen's test to demonstrate collateral blood supply to the hand.
- Brachial: Assess volume and character of pulses.
- Carotid: Remember palpate one at a time. In an elderly person with a rate of around 40 bpm don't assess carotids, as vagal stimulation may precipitate asystole!
- Abdominal aorta: In AAA there will be an expanding pulsation.
- Femorals: Assess for radio-femoral delay, which may indicate coarctation of the aorta.
- Popliteal: Assess for popliteal aneurysm.
- Dorsalis pedis and posterior tibial (only one needs to be present to mean there is circulation to the foot).
- Check sensation: This does not need to be a full neurological assessment; gross examination will identify paraesthesia in an emergency.
- Check the capillary refill time.

> **MICRO-facts**
>
> The radial pulse disappears when systolic BP is <70 mmHg.
> The femoral pulse disappears when systolic BP is <50 mmHg.

8.8.4 AUSCULTATION

- Listen for bruits, which indicate narrowing of the vessels.
  - In severe narrowing/occlusion there will not be a bruit, as there is no flow.
- Auscultate the carotids, aorta, femoral and subclavian arteries.

8.8.5 SPECIAL TESTS

- Blood pressure: This should be checked in both arms to look for asymmetry.
- Buerger's test:

- With the patient supine, elevate both legs to 45° and observe for pallor of the feet, indicating ischaemia. The poorer the arterial supply, the lower the angle at which pallor occurs.
- Next sit the patient with the legs hanging over the edge of the bed. As flow returns to the feet the colour will change from pale → blue (deoxygenated blood) → red (due to reactive hyperaemia).

- Ankle brachial pressure index (ABPI): This is the ratio of the ankle systolic pressure to the brachial systolic pressure. It is performed using a Doppler probe and blood pressure cuff (see Figure 8.9).

MICRO-facts

ABPI scores:
Normal: 1–1.2.
Claudication: 0.9–0.6.
Rest pain: 0.6–0.3.
Gangrene: <0.3.

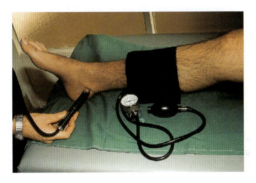

Figure 8.9 Measuring the ankle brachial pressure index (ABPI). (From: *Browse's Introduction to the Investigation and Management of Surgical Disease*, Figure 11.1, p. 235.)

8.9 THE DIABETIC FOOT

8.9.1 EPIDEMIOLOGY

- Diabetes is common, with 2.9 million people (4.45% of the population) diagnosed with the condition in the UK.
- Diabetics are 15 times more likely to undergo major lower limb amputation than non-diabetics.

8.9.2 AETIOLOGY

- See Figure 8.10.

General surgery

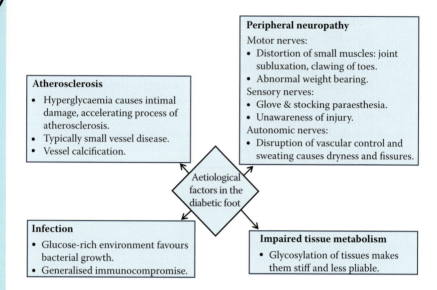

Atherosclerosis
- Hyperglycaemia causes intimal damage, accelerating process of atherosclerosis.
- Typically small vessel disease.
- Vessel calcification.

Peripheral neuropathy
Motor nerves:
- Distortion of small muscles: joint subluxation, clawing of toes.
- Abnormal weight bearing.
Sensory nerves:
- Glove & stocking paraesthesia.
- Unawareness of injury.
Autonomic nerves:
- Disruption of vascular control and sweating causes dryness and fissures.

Aetiological factors in the diabetic foot

Infection
- Glucose-rich environment favours bacterial growth.
- Generalised immunocompromise.

Impaired tissue metabolism
- Glycosylation of tissues makes them stiff and less pliable.

Figure 8.10 Aetiology of the diabetic foot.

MICRO-facts

Peripheral vascular disease commonly affects the below-knee trifurcation vessels in diabetics, giving rise to highly calcified arteries that may cause falsely elevated ABPI results (>1.0).

MICRO-facts

Risk factors for diabetic foot ulceration:
- Sensory neuropathy.
- Altered foot shape.
- Ill-fitting shoes.
- Previous ulceration.
- Peripheral vascular disease.
- Increasing age.
- Visual impairment.
- Living alone.

8.9.3 CLINICAL FEATURES

- The most common endpoint of diabetic vascular complications is foot ulceration.
  - May be purely neuropathic (~45–60%), purely ischaemic (~10%) or a mixture of the two (~25–45%) (see Table 8.1).

Infection

- Usually localised with pus and inflammation.
  - May be infection of existing ulcer or isolated (e.g. paronychia).

Table 8.1 Comparison between neuropathic and ischaemic ulcers.

CHARACTERISTICS	NEUROPATHIC	ISCHAEMIC
General features	Warm, dry foot. Bounding pulses. Distended veins. Sensory loss (pain and temperature). Painless necrosis of toes. Charcot's joint (painless, disorganised joint). Loss of foot arches.	Cool foot. Absent/reduced pulses. Painful ulcers. Wet or dry gangrene. Claudication. Rest pain.
Common sites for ulcers	Soles of the feet.	Heel. Malleoli. Head of fifth metatarsal. Tips of toes. Between the toes. Ball of the foot.
Ulcer appearance	Punched-out lesion surrounded by a ridge of calloused skin.	Looks like a poorly healed wound or a punched-out lesion with no surrounding callus.
Cause of ulceration	Repetitive or isolated trauma with lack of sensation.	Minor trauma.

- May lead to 'wet' gangrene (with pus and other exudate).
- Usually polymicrobial causation.
- May lead to osteomyelitis.

> **MICRO-facts**
>
> The punched-out appearance is due to rapid death and full-thickness sloughing of skin without successful attempts at repair, leaving a vertical edge. It is therefore seen in both neuropathic and ischaemic ulcers.

8.9.4 DIAGNOSIS

Bloods

- FBC to look for raised white cell count (WCC) when infected ulcers are suspected.
- U&E (often concomitant renal impairment).
- Cultures to guide antibiotic therapy if infected ulceration.
- ABPIs (see Section 8.8.5).
- Consider angiography if an ischaemic element is suspected.
- Perform plain x-rays of infected feet to rule out underlying osteomyelitis.

8.9.5 MANAGEMENT

General measures

- Regular inspection.
- Avoid potential damage:
  - Keep away from heat.
  - Do not walk barefoot.
- Pressure relief:
  - Appropriate, wide-fitting footwear.
- Chiropody:
  - Regular callus debridement.
  - Attention to nail care.

Best medical management

- Good glycaemic control.
- Anti-platelet, e.g. aspirin.
- Statin.

Assessment of ulcer type and aetiology

- Angiography if appropriate.
  - Consider revascularisation.
- Amputation.
  - Particularly common in patients who have underlying osteomyelitis.
  - Minor (digit/ray/forefoot) vs. major amputation (AKA/BKA) (Figure 8.11).
    - Minor amputations are rarely successful in ischaemic and neuroischaemic feet, as healing is poor due to inadequate blood supply.

Control infection

- Common causative organisms are Gram-positive aerobes in ~60%.
- Initial broad-spectrum (followed by targeted) antibiotic therapy.
- Surgical incision and drainage or debridement.
- Consider amputation.

8.10 VARICOSE VEINS

8.10.1 DEFINITION

- Varicose veins are elongated, dilated, often tortuous veins with incompetent valves (Figure 8.12).

8.10.2 EPIDEMIOLOGY

- They affect ~20% of the UK's population.
- Can be familial.

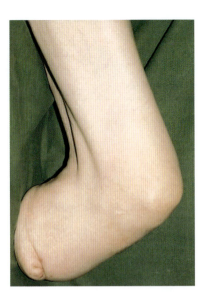

Figure 8.11 Below-knee amputation. (From: *Bailey & Love's Short Practice of Surgery, 26th Edition*, Figure 53.36, p. 917.)

Superficial system   Deep system

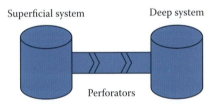

Perforators

Figure 8.12 The superficial and deep venous systems are connected at multiple sites via valved perforator veins.

8.10.3 CLASSIFICATION

Primary (most common)

- Primary degeneration of the valve annulus and leaflets (primary valve failure)
- Vein wall laxity, leading to widening of the valve commissures and incompetence (secondary valve failure).

Secondary

- Venous outflow obstruction.
  - E.g. pregnancy, fibroids, ovarian cysts, abdominal lymphadenopathy, pelvic cancer, iliac vein thrombosis, retroperitoneal fibrosis.
- Valve destruction.
  - E.g. DVT.

General surgery

> ### MICRO-facts
> N.B. It is necessary to ensure the deep venous system is functioning prior to surgical disconnection, because if it is non-functioning (e.g. in occlusive DVT) there is no alternative effective path of venous return.

8.10.4 CLINICAL FEATURES

Cosmetic
- Unsightly

Symptomatic
- Pain, discomfort or heaviness (worse on standing).
- Swelling/oedema.
- Nocturnal cramps.

Complications
- Ulceration.
- Bleeding.
- Phlebitis.
- Lipodermatosclerosis:
  - Eczema, itch, fat necrosis, pigmentation.

8.10.5 DIAGNOSIS

- Colour-coded duplex allows definition of anatomy and source of incompetence. It may also be used to assess the deep system.
- Venography: Varicosities may be marked with US guidance to aid surgery.
- Also see Section 8.11.

8.10.6 MANAGEMENT

Conservative
- Reassurance.
- Graduated compression stockings.
  - Problems with poor compliance.

Surgery
- Type of surgery varies as indicated by the outcome of clinical examination and duplex scan.
- E.g. ligation of the SFJ or SPJ with stripping and avulsions.
  - The incompetent vein is tied off and removed, and tributary veins are avulsed through small incisions over each vein.
  - Veins should be carefully marked pre-operatively.
    - Incisions should be placed away from ink to avoid tattooing.

Sclerotherapy

- Foam sclerosant is injected via a cannula under US guidance.
  - Not recommended for patients on oral contraceptive pill or hormone replacement therapy.
- Complications include:
  - Allergy, skin ulceration, phlebitis, pigmentation, nerve injury.

Endovenous laser ablation (EVLA)

- Uses a laser fibre passed into the vein under US guidance.
- Local anaesthetic is used before activation and withdrawal.

MICRO-print

Indications for the surgical treatment of varicose veins have become more stringent on account of their cosmetic nature and cost implications. It is now mostly restricted to patients with complications including haemorrhage, ulceration and thrombophlebitis.

8.11 HOW TO EXAMINE VARICOSE VEINS

- Varicose veins are common in clinical exams but are becoming less common in surgical outpatients due to the strict criteria for surgical intervention.
- Patients should be examined without socks or trousers, mandating privacy to maintain dignity.
- As always, ask permission before examining and ensure a chaperone is present.
- Start the examination in a standing position.

8.11.1 INSPECTION

- Examine the main distribution:
  - Medial thigh suggests long saphenous vein.
  - Posterior and lateral calf suggests short saphenous vein.
- Look for signs of complications or causation:
  - Oedema, lipodermatosclerosis, eczema, ulcers (usually over the medial malleolus.
  - Check for abdominal masses or pregnancy.

8.11.2 PALPATION

Tap test

- Place one hand on a prominent lower varicosity and use the other hand to gently tap downward over the vein from the SFJ.
- In a normal vein the impulse would be interrupted by competent valves; however in varicose veins you will feel the impulse further down the leg.

General surgery

Handheld doppler

- Holding the Doppler probe over the SFJ or SPJ, apply firm calf compression and listen for the resulting reflux signal.
  - A signal > 1–2 seconds suggests incompetence.

Tourniquet test

- Ask the patient to lie on the examination couch and elevate the leg, emptying the veins. Maintaining this position, apply a tourniquet over the SFJ before asking the patient to stand.
- Slowly release the tourniquet and observe the direction of filling:
  - If they fill rapidly from above, the SFJ is incompetent.
  - If they fill slowly from below with the tourniquet still applied, an incompetent perforator may be the cause.
- Examine for a saphenavarix at the SFJ by feeling for a swelling with a cough impulse.
- Ensure there are palpable foot pulses.

8.12 CAROTID DISEASE

8.12.1 EPIDEMIOLOGY

- Stroke disease is the third most common cause of death in the UK after myocardial infarction and cancer.
- Incidence of 2 per 1000 population in the UK.
- Approximately 30% of cerebrovascular accidents (CVAs) are due to carotid disease.

8.12.2 PATHOLOGY

- Atherosclerosis at the origin of the internal carotid artery (ICA), leading to stenosis.
- Unstable plaques may be a source of emboli to the cerebral circulation.
- The risk of CVA following a transient ischaemic attack (TIA) is 12–17% in the first year.
  - 20% of which occur within the first month.

> **MICRO-facts**
>
> Carotid bruits are audible in ~12% of patients over 60 years of age but bear no correlation to the degree of stenosis.

8.12.3 CLINICAL FEATURES

Asymptomatic

- May be an incidental finding:
  - On auscultation.

- On imaging for contralateral symptomatic disease.
- During workup for coronary surgery.

Amaurosis fugax

- This is transient loss of vision in one eye, described as a 'curtain coming down' across the vision, usually lasting a few minutes.
- It is ipsilateral.

TIA

- Transient loss of sensory or motor function, usually lasting a few minutes but always less than 24 hours.
- The contralateral side is affected.

CVA

- Neurological deficit lasting longer than 24 hours that may evolve over days, with progressive symptoms.

8.12.4 DIAGNOSIS

- All patients who suffer a TIA (including amaurosis) or non-disabling stroke should be investigated for treatable carotid disease.
- Duplex scan is the initial screening test, as it is non-invasive and has a high sensitivity for lesions with >50% stenosis.
- Magnetic resonance angiography (MRA) is more sensitive but is more expensive and may cause claustrophobia.
- Conventional angiography is invasive and carries a risk of embolic stroke (Figure 8.13).

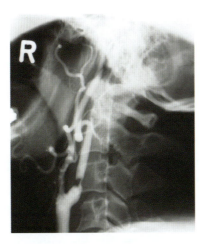

Figure 8.13 Carotid angiogram showing a tight stenosis. (From: *Browse's Introduction to the Investigation and Management of Surgical Disease*, Figure 11.31, p. 265.)

8.12.5 MANAGEMENT

- Management is summarised in Figure 8.14.
- Stenoses are considered significant at 70%.
- Best medical therapy:
  - Includes lifestyle advice, e.g. smoking cessation, regular physical activity, dietary changes.
  - Control hypertension and diabetes.
  - Anti-platelet therapy:
    - Low-dose aspirin ± dipyridamole, ticlopidine or clopidogrel.
  - Statin.

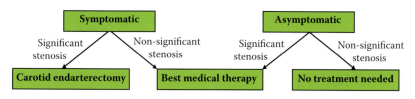

Figure 8.14 Management of carotid artery disease.

Carotid endarterectomy (CEA)

- This involves surgical removal of the stenotic plaque, aiming to prevent stroke.
- The procedure itself carries a small but significant risk of causing a stroke (approximately 2–4%).

Angioplasty and stenting

- Usually reserved for hostile necks (e.g. previous surgery or radiotherapy).

MICRO-print
- European and American trials have demonstrated a benefit of CEA in 70–99% stenoses with significantly lower risk of stroke or death at 2–3 years.
- However, no added benefit was found in patients with mild (0–29%) or moderate (30–69%) stenosis compared to best medical management alone.

MICRO-reference
ECST: European Carotid Surgery Trial. *Lancet* 1998; 351(9113): 1379–1387.
NASCET: North American Symptomatic Carotid Endarterectomy Trial. *Journal of Neurosurgery* 1995; 83(5): 778–782.

9.1 HOW TO EXAMINE THE MALE GENITALIA

- Although a separate specialty, urological presentations do form part of the general surgical emergency take. For this reason, we have covered acute urological conditions that may present during a general surgical on-call but have not dealt with elective urology.
- Wash hands in warm water and don gloves.
- Introduce self and obtain consent from the patient.
- Ensure curtains are closed to maintain patient dignity.
- Ask patient to lie on a couch, exposed from umbilicus to midway down the thigh.
- A chaperone must always be present for this examination.

9.1.1 INSPECTION

- Look for any obvious swelling, erythema or rashes.
- Note the secondary sexual characteristics (e.g. hair distribution).
- Assess cough, looking for evidence of herniae and cremasteric reflex.

Penis

- Inspect glans and shaft for warts, rashes or colour changes.

Scrotum

- Inspect for redness, swelling, ulcers or sebaceous cysts (common).
- Lift and inspect the posterior aspect of the scrotum as scrotal cancer (rare) most frequently presents as an ulcer here.

9.1.2 PALPATION

Penis

- Retract the foreskin to check for adhesions or phimosis.
  - Always draw foreskin back over the glans after examination to prevent occurrence of paraphimosis (see Section 9.10).
- Check the position of the urethral opening.
- Palpate/milk urethra and observe for any discharge.

Scrotum

- Check for presence of both testes in scrotum.
- Assess size and symmetry of testes.
- Palpate bimanually to examine for any lumps or asymmetry.
- If a lump is present use the three-question approach (see Figure 9.1).
- Note any tenderness of testes or epididymis.
- Palpate the vas deferens at the posteromedial aspect of the scrotal neck.
- Ask the patient to stand to identify if a varicocele is present.

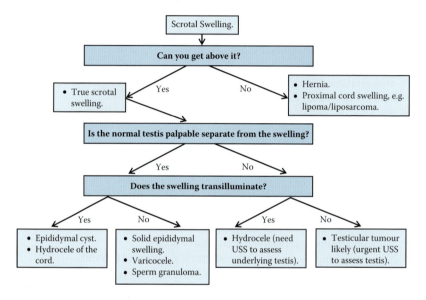

Figure 9.1 Three-question approach to examination of a scrotal swelling.

9.2 TESTICULAR TORSION

9.2.1 DEFINITION

- Testicular torsion is an acutely painful scrotum caused by the testis twisting on its cord structures.

9.2.2 EPIDEMIOLOGY

- Peak incidence is from adolescence to the third decade.

9.2.3 AETIOLOGY

- Congenital anatomical variant: The testicle lies horizontally; the 'bell clapper' lie.

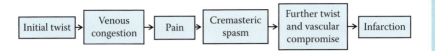

Figure 9.2 Pathological process in testicular torsion.

- Commonly occurs at night whilst in bed.
- See Figure 9.2.

9.2.4 CLINICAL FEATURES

- Sudden onset of severe scrotal pain.
- May have a history of similar, shorter-lived episodes with spontaneous resolution.
- Nausea and vomiting.
- Poorly localised lateralising lower abdominal pain (due to embryological nerve supply prior to descent of testicle into the scrotum).
- On examination:
  - High-riding testis.
  - Firm swelling above and posterior to the testis (torted cord).
  - Swollen, firm, tender testicle.
  - Extreme tenderness on examination.
  - Absence of ipsilateral cremasteric reflex.

9.2.5 INVESTIGATIONS

- If the history is short (e.g. presentation is within 24 hours of onset of pain), and torsion is suspected, investigations are inappropriate, as this is a surgical emergency.
- If the history is longer (e.g. over 24 hours from onset of pain), Doppler ultrasound scan (USS) may help differentiate from other causes (e.g. epidydimo-orchitis, testicular tumour).

MICRO-facts

When in doubt regarding a diagnosis of acute scrotum, urgent scrotal exploration should be performed.

9.2.6 MANAGEMENT

- Urgent surgical exploration of all suspected cases of testicular torsion is indicated, as irreversible testicular damage occurs within 6 hours of onset.

General surgery

Surgical procedure

- The scrotum is entered via a midline raphe incision.
- The cord structures are carefully de-torted.
- Assess if colour returns (Figure 9.3).

> **MICRO-print**
>
> Tip for surgeons intra-operatively to assess if the testis is viable: if in doubt, wrap the testicle in warm saline packs if dusky and leave for 5–10 minutes as colour may return. Also useful is a stab incision in the tunica albuginea to assess for bleeding.

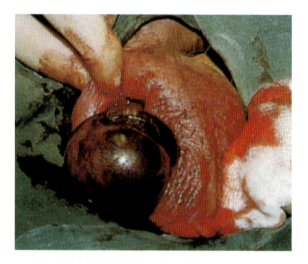

Figure 9.3 Surgical exploration reveals a torted testis. The tense, dark colour seen here indicates that this testis is unlikely to be salvageable. (From: *Illustrated Clinical Anatomy*, 2nd Edition., Figure 5.15, p. 82.)

- If viable, three-point fixation of the testis is performed using non-absorbable suture (orchidopexy).
- The contralateral testis should be fixed in the same way.
- If non-viable, the testis should be excised (orchidectomy) and the contralateral testis fixed to prevent subsequent torsion.
    - For this reason, all cases of scrotal exploration for presumed torsion must be consented for orchidectomy.

9.2.7 COMPLICATIONS

- Patient may experience reduced fertility in the future (even after surgical fixation).
- The testis, if partially ischaemic, may atrophy.

General surgery

> ## MICRO-facts
>
> Torsion of testicular appendage:
> - Torsion of one of the embryological remnants—either the testicular appendix (hydatid of Morgagni) or epididymal appendix.
> - Presentation mimics testicular torsion so is hard to distinguish.
> - 'Blue dot sign'—dark blue swelling in scrotum seen through the skin.
> - Management involves excision of affected appendage only.

9.3 EPIDIDYMO-ORCHITIS

9.3.1 EPIDEMIOLOGY

- Epididymo-orchitis has two peaks of incidence:
    - young adults;
    - over 50 years.

9.3.2 AETIOLOGY

- Commonly caused by STIs in the younger age group (e.g. *Chlamydia trachomatis*, *N. gonorrhoea*).
- The gut commensals are often the cause in older patients due to bladder outflow obstruction and urinary tract instrumentation.
- Mumps is an important cause of orchitis and may lead to testicular atrophy.

9.3.3 CLINICAL FEATURES

- Gradual onset of testicular pain over days-hours.
- Tender epididymis and testicle.
- Cremaster reflex is maintained.
- Positive Prehn's sign (relief of pain on scrotal elevation).
- Dysuria and urethral discharge may occur.

9.3.4 INVESTIGATIONS

- Full blood count (FBC) may show a raised white cell count (WCC).
- Urinalysis may reveal a pyuria.

9.3.5 MANAGEMENT

- This is with antibiotics.
    - If STI is suspected refer to genito-urinary medicine (GUM), as contact tracing may be needed.
    - In older men with benign prostatic obstruction a prolonged course of quinolone antibiotic (e.g. ciprofloxacin) is first-line treatment.

9.4 LOWER URINARY TRACT INFECTION (PYELONEPHRITIS)

9.4.1 EPIDEMIOLOGY

- Common in women, particularly during reproductive years.
    - In men, urinary tract infection (UTI) is often associated with underlying pathology (e.g. anatomical variant, bladder outflow obstruction).
    - In the elderly, recurrent UTI may be a manifestation of urothelial cancer.

MICRO-facts

Risk factors for UTI:
- Sexual activity.
- Pregnancy.
- Urinary tract malformation.
- Urinary tract obstruction.
- Stone disease.
- Bladder diverticula.
- Spinal injury.
- Trauma.
- Diabetes mellitus.
- Immunosuppression.

- Incidence of ~5% per year, accounting for 1–2% of primary care patients.
- UTI is an important cause of morbidity, especially in the elderly.

9.4.2 AETIOLOGY

- Cystitis occurs when bacteria track up the urethra into the bladder.
    - This is more common in women as the urethra is shorter and it ends on the perineum, making it possible to transfer organisms from the perineum to the end of the urethra during intercourse.
    - In men it may occur with incomplete bladder emptying associated with benign prostatic obstruction.
    - It is more common in diabetics, as glucosuria aids bacteria growth.
    - Bacteria causing cystitis are usually gut commensals (Gram-negative bacteria), e.g. *E. coli*, *Proteus mirabilis*, *Klebsiella*, *Enterococcus faecali*.

9.4.3 CLINICAL FEATURES

- Dysuria is a common symptom.
- Suprapubic pain or discomfort.
- Frequency of micturition.
- Frank haematuria may also occur.

9.4.4 INVESTIGATIONS

- UTI in males, children or if severe/recurrent all warrant further investigation.
- Urinalysis may reveal haematuria, nitrites, proteinuria and leucocytes on dipstick.
- Urine should be sent for MC&S to guide antibiotic therapy.

Bloods

- FBC may reveal raised WCC, particularly in pyelonephritis.
- U&E to assess kidney function and hydration status.
- USS of the urinary tract to look for a large residual volume following micturition.
- Cystoscopy in selected cases (e.g. men).

9.4.5 MANAGEMENT

- This is with antibiotics and varies with the causative organism, but trimethoprim, co-amoxiclav, cephalexin and nitrofurantoin may be used.

9.4.6 PROGNOSIS/COMPLICATIONS

- Women who have had a lower UTI are likely to have another. This may be minimised by the following general advice:
    - adequate oral hydration with water;
    - regular voiding;
    - voiding after intercourse;
    - avoiding the use of chemicals in baths (e.g. bubble bath);
    - cotton underwear (avoid nylon);
    - avoiding constipation.
  - Prophylactic antibiotics are given for frequent recurrences, but this is usually commenced by specialists.

9.5 UPPER UTI (PYELONEPHRITIS)

9.5.1 AETIOLOGY

- Pyelonephritis may occur due to ascending infection from the bladder or haematogenous spread to the kidney.
  - It is usually a one-off event.

9.5.2 CLINICAL FEATURES

- May occur with the symptoms of cystitis.
- There is loin pain and tenderness.

- Patients are severely unwell with systemic features (e.g. pyrexia and tachycardia).
- If severe, rigors may occur.

9.5.3 INVESTIGATIONS

- Urinalysis may reveal haematuria, nitrites, proteinuria and leucocytes on dipstick.
- Urine for MC&S to guide antibiotic therapy.

Bloods

- FBC may reveal raised WCC, particularly in pyelonephritis.
- U&E to assess kidney function and hydration status.
- Blood cultures should be sent.
- USS to assess for dilation of the ureters and pelvis.
- Abdominal x-ray (AXR) may be used to exclude a stone.
- Intravenous urogram (IVU) in recurrent pyelonephritis.
- Computed tomography (CT) if stones are suspected.

9.5.4 MANAGEMENT

- Management is with antibiotics.
  - This varies as to the causative organism, but in general cefuroxime or gentamicin (IV initially until sensitivities are available).

9.5.5 COMPLICATIONS

- Recurrent renal infection is unusual in an adult in the absence of stone disease.
- In childhood it may cause nephron loss and renal scarring, leading to cortical thinning, pitted external surface, and reduced size and renal function.

9.6 FOURNIER'S GANGRENE

- This is a form of necrotising fasciitis of the male genitalia and surrounding areas, typically caused by *Pseudomonas*, β-haemolytic streptococci, *E. coli* and *Clostridium*. It is rare and constitutes a surgical emergency.
- Without urgent debridement the mortality of the condition exceeds 90%.

MICRO-facts

Fournier's gangrene:
- Characterised by crepitus in an infected perineum.
- If you ever diagnose Fournier's gangrene you must act quickly. It is a urological emergency and requires **immediate** surgical debridement. Death can occur in hours and the overall mortality rate is high.

General surgery

9.7 UROLITHIASIS

9.7.1 EPIDEMIOLOGY

- 1 in 10 lifetime risk of stone disease.
- M:F 3:1.
- Peak age of presentation is 20–50 years.
- Commonest reason for an emergency urological admission.
- Peak time for presentation is in the summer months due to dehydration.

9.7.2 AETIOLOGY

- Many factors are known to play a role in stone development (Table 9.1).

Dietary oxalate

- E.g. chocolate, tea, rhubarb, spinach.

Hydration

- Stones are more likely to form if the patient is dehydrated.

Drugs

- Loop diuretics, chemotherapy agents, thiazides, allopurinol and indinavir.

Table 9.1 Types of urinary tract stones.

TYPES OF STONE	FREQUENCY	FACTS
Calcium stones	75%	May be calcium oxalate or phosphate stones. Usually small stones, but often sharp and may cause bleeding. Often idiopathic.
Triple phosphate stones (struvite)	15%	Mixture of magnesium, ammonium and calcium phosphate stones. May form staghorn calculi, often occur during chronic infection.
Uric acid stones	5%	Occur as a consequence of high uric acid levels. More common in gout and following chemotherapy for leukaemias and myeloproliferative disorders. Often radiolucent.
Cysteine	2–3%	Rare, occur in raised cysteine usually due to metabolic abnormalities. Can be radiolucent.
Xanthine and purine stones	1–2%	Rare. Due to inborn errors of metabolism.

Hypercalciurua and hypercalcaemia

- Hyperparathyroidism, following orthopaedic procedures, malignancy, increased vitamin D.

Infection

- Some organisms increase stone formation, e.g. *Proteus mirabilis* which produces urease and therefore increases urinary uric acid concentration by urea splitting.
- Metabolic and congenital urinary tract problems also increase the risk of stones.
- Stones may occur anywhere from the collecting ducts to the bladder.

> ## MICRO-facts
> Definitions:
> - **Hydronephrosis =** dilatation of the collecting system.
> - **Hydroureter =** dilatation of the ureter.
> - **Pyonephrosis =** an infected hydronephrosis.

9.7.3 CLINICAL FEATURES

Renal stones

- Can remain asymptomatic.
- Microscopic haematuria is the commonest presentation.
- Typically recurrent, dull loin pain.
- Often associated with infective symptoms.

Ureteric stones

- Present with ureteric colic. This is a severe pain that classically radiates from the loin to groin (due to the nerve supply of the ureter).
- The patient cannot get comfortable and is often writhing in pain.
- If the stone passes to the distal ureter, then urinary frequency and dysuria may occur.
- There is usually associated nausea, vomiting, sweating and tachycardia.
- The pain is usually continuous, with fluctuations in severity.
- Occasionally associated with macroscopic haematuria.

Bladder stones

- Often asymptomatic, but may cause suprapubic pain and terminal haematuria.
- They may cause retention of urine if blocking the urethra.
- Infection may occur along with the stone at any level of the urinary tract.

9.7.4 INVESTIGATIONS

- Urinalysis: 80% will have non-visible haematuria.
- MSU to detect concomitant infection.

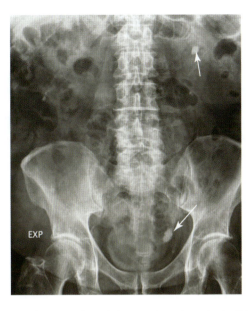

Figure 9.4 X-ray KUB showing a large left ureteric and renal calculi (arrows). (From: *Browse's Introduction to the Investigation and Management of Surgical Disease*, Figure 20.3, p. 505.)

- Bloods: FBC, U&E, serum calcium, phosphate and uric acid.
- Plain x-ray will often miss ureteric stones, despite the fact that around ~90% of stones are radio-opaque (Figure 9.4).
- Non-contrast CT scan is the gold standard for diagnosing stones.
  - CT will also exclude other causes of pain, e.g. appendicitis or AAA.
- Intravenous urogram (IVU) may be used, though this is being replaced by CT.
- Ultrasound may be used to detect secondary hydronephrosis if there is a chance the patient is pregnant, but will not show the stone.

9.7.5 MANAGEMENT

- Ensure adequate analgesia: e.g. morphine or diclofenac (beware non-steroidal anti-inflammatory drugs (NSAIDs) in renal impairment).
- Encourage oral fluid intake and prescribe intravenous infusion (IVI) if signs of dehydration (due to persistent vomiting).
- Alpha-blockers (e.g. tamsulosin) may be given in stones in the lower 1/3 of the ureter to relax the smooth muscle.
  - This relieves pain and may facilitate passage but is an un-licensed indication.
- Observe the patient for sepsis.
  - Urgent nephrostomy is indicated in patients with fever and a tender kidney.

- Small stones (<6 mm) are managed conservatively.
  - 80% of stones >8 mm will not pass spontaneously and will require intervention.
  - 90% of stones <6 mm will pass spontaneously, requiring no intervention.

> ### MICRO-facts
>
> **Indications for intervention:** Sepsis, solitary kidney with renal impairment, unremitting pain, profession (pilots cannot fly with a known ureteric stone).

Management of larger ureteric stones

- Extracorporeal shockwave lithotripsy (ESWL).
  - This is targeted energy at the stone to fragment it to allow it to pass.
  - Stone must be visible on x-ray or US.
  - They may need multiple treatments.
  - It is contra-indicated in pregnancy, coagulopathy and calcified AAA.
- Rigid ureteroscopy:
  - Direct visualisation and fragmentation of stones using laser or US.
- Percutaneous nephrolithotomy for renal stones:
  - A nephroscope is passed into the kidney (as in a nephrostomy), and then the stone is fragmented and fragments extracted.
- Open surgery is almost never required in modern practice.

9.7.6 COMPLICATIONS

Hydronephrosis

- Due to impaction of the stone.

Superimposed infection in obstruction

- This is a urological emergency—the kidney requires decompression to save future function.
  - IV antibiotics should be administered.
  - Emergency nephrostomy is a radiological procedure where a tube is inserted into the renal pelvis or ureter, allowing urine drainage.
  - Double J stents may be used in patients where nephrostomy is not available or appropriate (e.g. bleeding diathesis).
- Up to 50% have recurrent stones in 5 years.
  - Encourage high fluid intake.
  - Treat UTIs early.
  - In idiopathic hypercalciuria give thiazide diuretic to ↓ calcium excretion.
  - Reduce oxalate intake.
  - Alkalinise urine in uric acid stones.

> **MICRO-case**
>
> A 55-year-old male presents to the emergency department with severe left-sided loin pain that radiates to his groin. The pain is coming in waves and he cannot get comfortable. He feels feverish and unwell. He denies dysuria.
>
> On examination he is tender in his left renal angle and has a temperature of 38°C. His WCC is 18×10^9, U&E tests are normal and he has microscopic haematuria on urine dipstick.
>
> He is admitted, given IV fluids and IV antibiotics before undergoing non-contrast CT scanning, which confirms a 7-mm left PUJ stone with evidence of hydronephrosis and infection. Urgent nephrostomy insertion was carried out with immediate resolution of fever and pain.
>
> **Learning points:**
> - An infected, obstructed kidney is an emergency, requiring immediate intervention.
> - Irreversible renal deterioration can occur in an obstructed kidney in the presence of infection within 6 hours.
> - In a single obstructed kidney, there is often no deterioration in renal function blood tests as the contralateral kidney continues to function.

9.8 URINARY RETENTION

9.8.1 DEFINITION

- Urinary retention is the inability to pass urine and may be acute or chronic.
- Patients with acute urinary retention commonly present to the emergency general surgical take.
- Acute urinary retention is defined by the presence of severe suprapubic pain in association with a tender palpable bladder that is relieved completely and instantaneously on drainage of the bladder.
  - In contrast, chronic urinary retention with associated secondary UTI may present with discomfort, but not severe pain, and is not associated with immediate relief.

9.8.2 AETIOLOGY

- May be broadly classified as obstructive or detrusor failure (Figure 9.5).

9.8.3 CLINICAL FEATURES

Inability to pass urine

- Acute urinary retention is very painful and the retained urine volume is usually less than 1000 mL.
- Chronic urinary retention is painless, but may be associated with much higher retained urine volumes.

General surgery

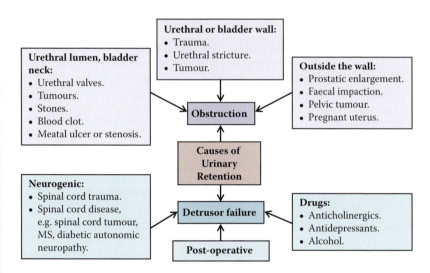

Figure 9.5 Causes of urinary retention.

> **MICRO-print**
> Post-operative urinary retention is very common in elderly men. A digital rectal examination should always be performed to exclude locally advanced prostate cancer. Most patients who fail a trial without catheter (TWOC) can be taught clean intermittent self-catheterisation (CISC). Resumption of spontaneous voiding occurs in the majority within 6 weeks.

- Other lower urinary tract symptoms (LUTSs) may have been present:
  - Poor stream, frequency and hesitancy.
- Symptoms of UTI may be present.

On examination

- An enlarged bladder will be palpable, often to the level of the umbilicus.
- PR examination may reveal an enlarged or abnormal prostate.
- In chronic retention, catheterisation usually drains clear urine initially, sometimes with terminal haematuria resulting from decompression.

9.8.4 DIAGNOSIS

- Urinary retention is a clinical diagnosis.
  - In obese patients, simple bladder scanning on the ward can be particularly helpful in aiding diagnosis.
- U&E should always be performed to ensure there is no renal impairment.
- USS to look for hydronephrosis and hydroureter caused by obstructive uropathy.

- Cystoscopy may be performed if there is haematuria or suspicion of a stricture (e.g. unable to insert urethral catheter).

> **MICRO-facts**
>
> Contra-indications to suprapubic catheterisation (SPC):
> - Lower midline scars.
> - Unable to palpate bladder.
> - History of bladder cancer.
> - Unexplained haematuria.

9.8.5 MANAGEMENT

- The immediate management of urinary retention should be urethral catheterisation.
  - If the urethral catheter will not pass, seek senior help.
    - The patient may require suprapubic catheterisation (SPC).
- Patients in acute urinary retention may require analgesia prior to catheterisation.
- If there is new renal impairment, IV fluid therapy should be commenced and the U&E repeated at 24 hours.
- The patients should be referred to the urology team on the post-take ward round for further investigation.

> **MICRO-case**
>
> An 80-year-old male who underwent bilateral hernia repairs is unable to pass urine post-operatively and is in significant pain. On examination he has a palpable, tender bladder. The on-call doctor inserts a urinary catheter and checks his U&E (which are normal). The next morning he undergoes TWOC, following which he successfully passes urine. He is discharged later that day.
>
> **Learning points:**
> - Most post-operative urinary retention will resolve within 24 hours.
> - U&E should be checked in all patients presenting with urinary retention.

9.9 FRANK HAEMATURIA

9.9.1 DEFINITION

- Haematuria is the passage of blood in the urine; it may be microscopic or macroscopic.
- Frank haematuria is a common presentation on the emergency surgical take and may present with associated acute urinary retention due to blood clots.

9.9.2 AETIOLOGY

- Depends on the level of pathology (Figure 9.6).

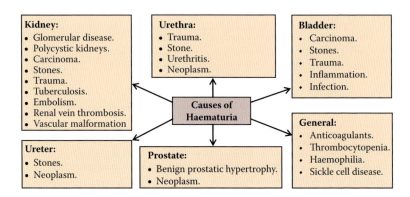

Figure 9.6 Causes of haematuria.

9.9.3 CLINICAL FEATURES

- The colour of frank haematuria may vary from rosé to dark blood with clots.
- Timing of blood in the urinary stream may give an indication of the bleeding site:
    - Early in the stream suggests a urethral or prostatic aetiology.
    - At the end of the stream is suggestive of trigonal or bladder neck pathology.
    - Blood throughout the stream suggests an upper urinary tract cause.
    - Urethral bleeding independent of urination suggests a urethral or prostatic lesion.
- The presence of pain may also suggest a cause:
    - Loin pain or ureteric colic may suggest a stone or renal tumour.
    - Suprapubic discomfort may suggest a bladder stone or UTI.
- On examination there may be a palpable kidney, bladder or prostate.

> **MICRO-facts**
>
> 20% of patients with macroscopic haematuria and <5% of patients with microscopic haematuria will have an underlying urological malignancy.

9.9.4 DIAGNOSIS

- In the acute setting all patients need a FBC, U&E, and clotting screen.
- Urine should be sent for microscopy and culture.
- If there is a suggestion of stone disease or renal impairment a USS or non-contrast CT of the renal tract is needed to exclude hydronephrosis.
- Flexible cystoscopy should also be arranged.

General surgery

9.9.5 MANAGEMENT

- Depends on the underlying cause.
- Patients with clot retention may require catheterisation and bladder irrigation.
- Analgesia for patients with clot colic.
- IV fluids for patients with associated renal impairment.
- Antibiotics for haematuria associated with UTI.
- Persistent haematuria may cause a drop in haemoglobin and so patients may rarely require transfusion.
- Patients with negative investigations can usually be reassured if the haematuria resolves spontaneously.

9.10 PARAPHYMOSIS

- Paraphymosis results from retraction of a tight foreskin. If it is not replaced, it causes constriction of the glans, leading to swelling and pain. As the oedema increases it becomes more difficult to reduce.

9.10.1 MANAGEMENT

- Conservative measures to aid reduction include:
  - Ice packs, direct pressure to reduce the oedema, sugar granules (osmotic effect).
- Invasive manoeuvres to aid reduction include:
  - Penile LA ring blocks, needle drainage of oedema fluid (multiple prick technique) under Emla™ cover.
- Elective circumcision at a later date should be considered in all patients to prevent recurrence.

9.11 PRIAPISM

9.11.1 DEFINITION

- Prolonged, painful erection that is not associated with sexual desire.

9.11.2 CAUSES

- Erectile dysfunction therapy, particularly if administered by intracorporeal injection.
- Haematological disease (due to hyperviscosity).
- Malignant infiltration.
- Neurological disease.
- Drugs (e.g. anti-hypertensives, anti-depressants).

General surgery

9.11.3 MANAGEMENT

- Conservative measures should be tried initially, including:
  - vigorous exercise (e.g. running up and down stairs);
  - cold baths and ice packs.
- Invasive manoeuvres (including needle aspiration, intracorporeal injection of an alpha-agonist and surgical intervention) should be undertaken by a urologist.

9.11.4 PROGNOSIS

- May lead to impotence if not treated (occurs in ~90% of priapism lasting > 24 hours).

9.12 HOW TO INSERT A URINARY CATHETER

9.12.1 OPENING

- Collect all necessary equipment.
- Introduce self and obtain consent from the patient.
- Ensure curtains are closed to maintain patient dignity.
- Put on apron and wash hands.

MICRO-print

Ch. or Charière gauge: Diameter of the catheter in mm [also called French (or Fr.) gauge].

    Foley: Catheter with self-retaining balloon.

    Coudé: 'Bent' like an elbow (to aid insertion around a large prostate).

    3-way: A triple-lumen catheter. One lumen allows bladder washout to be performed with sterile water, one lumen allows bladder drainage and the remaining lumen is used to inflate the self-retaining balloon.

MICRO-facts

Appropriate catheters:
- Simple urinary retention: Size 12–14 Ch. Foley.
- Chronic retention: Consider suprapubic catheter primarily.
- Clot retention: 20 Ch+ simplastic three-way catheter.
- Difficult insertion: Try Coudé 14–16 Ch.

9.12.2 PROCEDURE (MALE CATHETERISATION)

- It is important to practice aseptic technique and maintain a sterile field at all times.
- Open catheterisation pack and packaging of all other equipment into the sterile field of the catheter pack.

- Expose patient from umbilicus to mid-thigh level.
- Put on sterile gloves and create sterile patient field using sterile towels leaving the penis exposed.
- Using a swab to hold the penis, clean the urethral meatus with 0.9% saline-soaked cotton wool balls using single downward strokes (one cotton wool ball per stroke).
- Insert syringe containing anaesthetic gel into urethra holding the penis in a vertical position.
- Wait 3–5 minutes before continuing.
- Gently insert the catheter into urethra, making sure to avoid contact with genitalia to avoid contamination.
- Observe for urine flow to ensure that catheter is in bladder, and then advance catheter fully up to the bifurcation.
- Inflate balloon with the appropriate amount of 0.9% saline.
- Connect catheter-to-catheter bag.
- Replace foreskin to prevent occurrence of paraphimosis.
- Fix catheter to thigh with tape to reduce discomfort.

9.12.3 PROCEDURE (FEMALE CATHETERISATION)

- As for male catheterisation, except the left hand is used to part the labia in order to visualise the urethra.
    - In the obese or those with vaginal atrophy, position the index and middle finger of your left hand just behind the palpable urethral orifice to guide the tip of the advancing catheter upward into the urethra.

General surgery

10 Burns and trauma

10.1 ATLS™ PRINCIPLES

- Advanced Trauma Life Support (ATLS™) is an international, standardised method of assessing and managing trauma patients.
  - The premise of ATLS™ is to treat the greatest threat to life first.
  - This overview is not designed to replace the course!

10.1.1 PRIMARY SURVEY

- The initial assessment is known as the primary survey.
  - Life-threatening injuries are identified and treated.
  - Simultaneous commencement of resuscitation.
    - The level of resuscitation depends on the type of injury, e.g.:
      - Patients with significant head injury should have normotensive resuscitation, maintaining a systolic BP of 110 mmHg to prevent secondary brain injury.
      - In patients without head injury, hypotensive resuscitation is more common (to maintain a systolic BP of around 90 mmHg).
- The mnemonic ABCDE is used to remember the order in which problems should be addressed.
  - Occasionally in massive trauma situations catastrophic haemorrhage control may become the first priority before the usual airway and breathing assessments and is described as the <C>ABCDE approach.

10.1.2 A: AIRWAY MAINTENANCE (WITH CERVICAL SPINE PROTECTION)

- The airway should be assessed first to ascertain patency.
  - Look for:
    - foreign bodies;
    - fluid, e.g. blood or vomit;
    - facial, mandibular or tracheal/laryngeal fractures.
  - If the patient is able to talk, the airway is likely to be clear.
  - Patients with an altered level of consciousness may not be able to maintain their own airway.

      – Those with a Glasgow Coma Scale (GCS) (see Table 10.1) score of 8 or less usually require the placement of a definitive (i.e. an endotracheal tube) or surgical (i.e. cricothyroidotomy) airway.

- Initially the airway should be opened using the 'chin lift' or 'jaw thrust' manoeuvres.
- Airway adjuncts may be needed, such as:
  - oropharyngeal or nasopharyngeal airways;
  - suction devices.
- Care should be taken to avoid excessive movement of the cervical spine during assessment and management of the airway.
  - An unstable cervical spine injury should be suspected in all patients who have sustained a head injury or multi-system traumatic insult.
  - Protection of the spinal cord should be achieved with immobilisation devices until the C-spine is cleared of injury.
    - If immobilisation devices are temporarily removed the neck should be manually stabilised by a team member.

Table 10.1 Elements of the Glasgow Coma Scale.

	EYES	VERBAL	MOTOR
1	Does not open eyes.	Makes no sounds.	Makes no movements.
2	Opens eyes in response to painful stimuli.	Incomprehensible sounds.	Extension to painful stimuli (decerebrate response).
3	Opens eyes in response to voice.	Utters inappropriate words.	Abnormal flexion to painful stimuli (decorticate response).
4	Opens eyes spontaneously.	Confused, disoriented.	Flexion/withdrawal to painful stimuli.
5	N/A.	Oriented, converses normally.	Localises to painful stimuli.
6	N/A.	N/A.	Obeys commands.

10.1.3 B: BREATHING AND VENTILATION

- Ventilation requires adequate function of the lungs, chest wall and diaphragm. Each of these should be rapidly evaluated as part of B.
- The entire chest should be exposed to allow visual inspection of chest wall injuries, assessment of chest wall movement and auscultation of both lungs.
  - Assessment should concentrate on the identification and management of any condition that may cause an immediate threat to ventilation:
    - tension pneumothorax (see Section 10.3.2);

- – flail chest with pulmonary contusions (see Section 10.3.1);
- – massive haemothorax (see Section 10.3.3).
- High-flow oxygen should be commenced simultaneously at this stage.

10.1.4 C: CIRCULATION WITH HAEMORRHAGE CONTROL

- Haemorrhage is the predominant cause of preventable post-injury deaths.
- Hypotension following trauma should be considered to be due to hypovolaemia from blood loss until proven otherwise.
  - Useful indicators of hypovolaemia include:
    - – Pulse (rate and rhythm): Tachycardia may be the first sign of hypovolaemia.
    - – Blood pressure—Significant blood loss with result in hypotension, but a low blood pressure may also be due to other causes.
    - – Skin colour: Hypovolaemic patients may appear grey and clammy with pale extremities.
    - – Level of consciousness: Cerebral perfusion may be impaired by loss of circulating blood volume, resulting in a reduced conscious level.
    - – However, conscious patients may also have sustained significant blood loss.
- Two large-bore intravenous lines should be inserted at this stage and 2 crystalloid solution should be given.
  - If there is no response, cross-matched type-specific blood, or O-negative if this is not available, should be commenced, depending on the degree of urgency.
- External haemorrhage should be identified and controlled using direct, manual pressure to the wound during the primary survey.
- Occult, life-threatening haemorrhage should be considered in all trauma patients and may occur in the following areas:
  - Chest, abdomen, retroperitoneum, pelvis, long bones.
- It is important to remember that surgical intervention may be required as part of C to establish haemorrhage control.

10.1.5 D: DISABILITY (NEUROLOGIC EVALUATION)

- This should establish the patient's conscious level (using the GCS; see Table 10.1), pupil size and reaction, lateralising signs and spinal cord injury level.
- Hypoglycaemia and drugs (including alcohol) may result in a reduced conscious level.
  - A BM should be taken at this stage to rule out hypoglycaemia.
- The Glasgow Coma Scale comprises three tests: eye, verbal and motor responses.
  - The lowest possible score is 3 (deep coma or death).
  - The highest is 15—a fully awake person.

General surgery

10.1.6 E: EXPOSURE/ENVIRONMENTAL CONTROL

- The patient should be completely undressed to allow full assessment of injuries.
- Following this he or she should be covered with blankets to prevent hypothermia.
  - In patients who arrive with hypothermia, warming blankets and warmed IV fluids may be used to correct their temperature.

10.1.7 SECONDARY SURVEY

- When the primary survey is completed, resuscitation should be well underway and the vital signs should be normalising.
  - Reassessment is key.
    - If there is no improvement in vital signs, assessment should begin again at ABCDE before moving on.
    - If there is subsequent deterioration during the secondary survey, a further primary survey should be commenced.
- The secondary survey is a comprehensive head-to-toe evaluation, including a complete history and full examination.
  - Specific areas that should not be forgotten include:
    - full spinal examination;
    - perineum, vagina and rectum;
    - back of the head;
    - limbs.
- Standard trauma x-rays (C-spine, chest and pelvis) are obtained.
- Full bloods, if not obtained during the primary survey, should be taken now, including full blood count (FBC), urea and electrolytes (U&E), liver function tests (LFTs), clotting screen, group and save or cross-match.
- An AMPLE history may be required from a family member in patients who are unconscious:
  - allergies;
  - medications;
  - past medical history;
  - last meal;
  - events related to the injury.

MICRO-references

Committee on Trauma, American College of Surgeons (2008). *ATLS: Advanced Trauma Life Support program for doctors* (8th ed.). Chicago: American College of Surgeons.

10.2 ABDOMINAL TRAUMA

- Surgery is necessary in:
  - ~10% blunt abdominal trauma;
  - ~40% stab wound victims;
  - ~95% of patients with gunshot wounds (GSWs).

MICRO-facts

Indications for consideration of immediate laparotomy in trauma patients:
- A GSW to the abdomen, particularly if haemodynamically unstable.
- A stab wound to the abdomen in a haemodynamically unstable patient.
- Clinical evidence of intra-abdominal bleeding (e.g. blunt abdominal injury, seat belt mark, increasing distension) in a haemodynamically unstable patient.
- Peritonitis.
- Recurrent hypotension despite adequate fluid resuscitation.
- Air under the diaphragm on imaging.
- Evidence of diaphragmatic injury on imaging.
- CT evidence of significant injury to an intra-abdominal viscus (e.g. splenic rupture).

10.2.1 HEPATIC TRAUMA

- Hepatic injuries are graded according to their severity, with I (one) being a small haematoma or capsular tear and VI being hepatic avulsion.
  - 80–90% of all hepatic injuries are grade I or II, requiring no operative intervention.
    - Patients undergoing conservative management require continual reassessment. This is not usually possible if they require operative intervention for other injuries.

Clinical features
- RUQ pain.
- Signs of hypovolaemic shock in severe injuries.

Non-operative management
- Continual reassessment and re-imaging.
- Correct clotting abnormalities.
- Blood transfusion if required.
- Angioembolisation may be attempted if available locally.
- Consider re-imaging and operative intervention if clinical deterioration.

10.2.2 SPLENIC TRAUMA

- Splenic injuries are graded from I to V, with I being a small haematoma or capsular tear and V being a completely shattered spleen.
- Clinical features:
  - LUQ pain.
    - There may be pain referred to the left shoulder tip (Kehr's sign).
  - Severe injuries may present with evidence of a haemorrhage that continues despite resuscitation.

MICRO-print

Secondary haemorrhage:

- Following the initial injury there may be a period of recovery lasting hours to days as bleeding is arrested (either by omentum or a clot) or a haematoma stops expanding.
- This is followed by dislodgement (of omentum or clot) or capsular rupture, resulting in a second, more profound bleed with collapse, shock and generalised abdominal pain.

Management

- Splenic injuries may be managed conservatively if the patient is stable.
  - Patients with high-grade splenic injuries should be observed closely for 48–72 hours due to the risk of secondary rupture.
- Indications for consideration of operative intervention:
  - >4-unit blood transfusion in 48 hours;
  - other intra-abdominal injuries;
  - continuing haemodynamic instability despite resuscitation.
- In severe injuries requiring surgical intervention, splenectomy is usually performed.

MICRO-print

Overwhelming post-splenectomy infection (OPSI):

- Patients following splenectomy are at risk of OPSI, which is rare but may be rapidly fatal.
  - Lifetime risk is approximately 5% in splenectomised patients.
- Responsible organisms are encapsulated organisms, e.g. *Streptococcus pneumonia*, *Haemophillus influenzae*, *Neisseria meningitidis*.
- Patients require vaccination against these organisms and long-term antibiotic prophylaxis (e.g. with penicillin V).

10.2.3 PERFORATED INTRA-ABDOMINAL VISCUS

Mechanisms
- Road traffic accident (RTA):
  - Compression injuries (e.g. from a seat belt in an RTA).
  - Rapid deceleration with shearing and rotational forces can lead to burst bowel and torn mesentery.
- Penetrating injuries (knife stab wounds, GSWs).

Clinical features
- Generalised abdominal pain.
- Rigid, tender, silent abdomen.
- Systemically unwell:
  - Tachycardia.
  - Tachypnoea.
  - Hypotension.
  - Pyrexia.

Management
- Evidence of a perforated intra-abdominal viscus is an indication for immediate laparotomy in the trauma setting.

10.2.4 DAMAGE CONTROL SURGERY (DCS)

Principles of DCS
- Control of haemorrhage.
- Prevention of contamination.
- Protection from further injury.
- Based on the reality that trauma patients are more likely to die from the physiological triad of coagulopathy, hypothermia and metabolic acidosis than anatomic injury.
- Initial procedure is therefore shortened so the patient can be transferred to a critical care department for correction of hypothermia and acidosis.
  - Following this, definitive surgical procedures may be carried out as required when the patient is more stable.

10.3 THORACIC TRAUMA

> ## MICRO-facts
> **Indications for chest drain insertion:** Compromise in ventilation due to the presence of one of the following in the thoracic cavity:
> - Air (pneumothorax).
> - Blood (haemothorax).
>
> *continued...*

General surgery

continued...

- Pus (empyema).
- Lymph (chylothorax).
- Fluid (effusion).

- Traumatic chest injuries cause 25% of trauma deaths in the UK.
- Less than 15% of all chest trauma patients require surgery.
- Blunt trauma (usually due to RTAs) is the most prevalent type in the UK.

10.3.1 FLAIL CHEST

- This is when there are two or more fractures in two or more adjacent ribs, causing a segment of the chest wall to lose bony continuity with the rest of the thoracic cage.

Clinical features

- Respiratory distress.
- Paradoxical chest wall movements.
- Hypoxia.
- Hypovolaemia.
- Crepitus over the ribs.

Management

- Respiratory support if required.
- Analgesia.
- Drainage of haemothorax if required.
- Operative stabilisation is rarely indicated.

Complications

- Atelectasis.
- Pneumonia.

10.3.2 TENSION PNEUMOTHORAX

- A pneumothorax is an abnormal collection of air or gas in the pleural space that separates the lung from the chest wall.
- A tension pneumothorax is caused when a one-way valve is formed by an area of damaged tissue so that the amount of air in the chest increases dramatically.
  - This results in respiratory and circulatory distress.

Clinical features

- Respiratory distress.
- Tracheal deviation away from the affected side.
- Unilaterally decreased breath sounds (on the affected side).

- Raised JVP.
- Pulseless electrical activity (PEA) cardiac arrest.

Management

- Immediate needle decompression.
  - In trauma in extremis a thoracostomy (chest wall incision into the pleural cavity) may be used instead.
- IV access.
- Chest drain insertion.

10.3.3 MASSIVE HAEMOTHORAX

- Defined as >1500 mL blood drained on the insertion of a chest drain.
- Usually a result of a penetrating injury.

Clinical features

- Hypovolaemic shock.
- Absent breath sounds and dull percussion note on the affected side.
- Evidence of a penetrating wound.

Management

- IV resuscitation.
- Chest drain insertion.
- Emergency thoracotomy is indicated for continuing loss:
  - >2000 mL drained immediately;
  - 200 mL/hour drained subsequently.

MICRO-facts

The classical trio of signs ($\uparrow$ JVP, $\downarrow$ BP and muffled heart sounds) is known as .

10.3.4 CARDIAC TAMPONADE

- This is an acute pericardial effusion causing pressure on the heart muscle.
- Most commonly a result of a stab wound from a knife in the UK.
- Usually injury to the left or right ventricle.

Clinical features

- Raised JVP.
- Hypotension.
- Muffled heart sounds.
- Increased JVP on inspiration (Kussmaul's sign).
- PEA cardiac arrest.
- Diagnosis may be confirmed by focussed assessment with sonography for trauma (FAST) scan.

Management

- Urgent pericardiocentesis.
  - This is diagnostic and therapeutic, as it allows decompression.
  - If there is clot formation, aspiration may not work leading to a false negative result.
- The alternative diagnostic procedure is a subxiphoid window (a surgical opening in the pericardium via a subxiphoid incision).
- Ultimately, treatment is by thoracotomy or sternotomy.

10.4 HEAD TRAUMA

10.4.1 AETIOLOGY

- Common causes include:
  - Falls.
    - May be secondary to alcohol excess, which is important when assessing the patient.
  - RTA.

> **MICRO-facts**
>
> See NICE guideline CG56, Head injury from 2007, for full guidance on the recommended triage, admission, monitoring and referral criteria.

10.4.2 DEFINITIONS

- Concussion: A transient loss of consciousness for hours with then apparent clinical recovery.
- Diffuse axonal injury: A radiological diagnosis. It is due to sudden forces applied to the head (e.g. sudden acceleration, deceleration or rotation), which leads to shearing of neurons at the grey-white interface, at the end of the myelin sheath. This has a poor outcome.

10.4.3 TYPES OF SKULL FRACTURE

- May be open (with overlying soft tissue injury) or closed.
- Depressed skull fractures require neurosurgical input.

> **MICRO-facts**
>
> Examine patients with head injuries for signs of basal skull fracture:
> - Panda eyes.
> - Subconjunctival haemorrhage.
> - Haemotympanum.
> - Battle's sign: bruising behind the ears.

10.4.4 TYPES OF BRAIN INJURY

Primary

- Injury to the brain directly due to the head injury.
  - E.g. contusion, diffuse axonal injury, brain haemorrhage.

Secondary

- Due to the effects of injury in general.
  - E.g. cerebral hypoxia due to hypovolaemia.

10.4.5 HAEMORRHAGE

Extradural

- Most often (but not exclusively) due to damage to the middle meningeal artery with temporal bone fractures.
- Usually follows blunt trauma.
- Clinical features:
  - Period of unconsciousness followed by a lucid period. Then falling GCS and signs of raised intracranial pressure (ICP) leading to (if not treated) death.

Acute subdural (Figure 10.1)

- Due to tearing of veins in the subdural space.
- Often follows a high-speed collision.

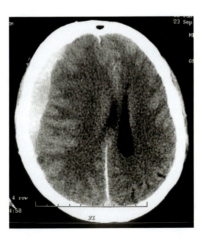

Figure 10.1 CT scan showing a right-sided acute subdural haematoma. Note the midline shift to the left. (From: *Bailey & Love's Short Practice of Surgery, 25th Edition*, Figure 23.8, p. 305.)

General surgery

- Clinical features:
  - Deterioration in consciousness within minutes of injury.
  - May be preceded by initial loss of consciousness, followed by a short lucid period.
  - Often accompanied by signs of raised ICP.

Chronic subdural

- Seen in the elderly due to increased risk of tearing veins due to age-related brain atrophy.
- Head injury may only have been very minor.
- Symptoms develop over days/weeks with focal deficits, headache and loss of consciousness.
- Asymptomatic chronic subdural haematomas are often managed conservatively with serial imaging.

Subarachnoid

- May occur following head injury or conversely may cause loss of consciousness prior to head injury.
- Seen in those with aneurysm disease, often as a first presentation.

Intraparenchymal

  - Commonly occur alongside diffuse axonal injury.
  - In children, may be due to non-accidental injury.
- All intracranial haemorrhage should be discussed with neurosurgical team and where appropriate, transferred to the neurosurgical unit for further treatment.
  - Definitive management may involve surgical evacuation of haematoma or clipping/coiling of aneurysms.

10.4.6 IMMEDIATE MANAGEMENT

- Remember ABC resuscitation: Ensure the brain is being oxygenated, which relies on a patent airway and adequate BP for perfusion (normotensive resuscitation).
- Immobilise C-spine and image significant head injuries.
  - Especially in polytrauma (e.g. RTA) or if associated with a fall to the ground.
- Assess brain injury as part of D in primary trauma survey.
  - Use GCS, pupillary response, baseline observations and don't forget glucose and collateral history.
  - Assess for skull damage and look for signs of CSF leak: rhinorrhoea, otorrhoea.
  - Involve anaesthetics early for opinion on ventilation and then ITU admission.
  - If GCS is <8, then the patient cannot protect his or her own airway.
- Early discussion with local neurosurgical unit.

MICRO-facts

Criteria for urgent CT in a head injury patient:

- GCS < 13 on initial assessment or < 15 at 2 hours post-injury.
- Suspected open or depressed skull fracture.
- Evidence of basal skull fracture (see micro-facts box above).
- More than one episode of vomiting.
- Post-traumatic seizure.
- Coagulopathy (e.g. current warfarin therapy) in the presence of amnesia or loss of consciousness.

10.4.7 OBSERVATION/MONITORING

- If in doubt, admit (especially if under the influence of alcohol) for 24 hours of observation.
- Regular neuro-observations (including GCS):
  - Drop in consciousness will occur prior to any physical sign changes.
- Monitor baseline observations:
  - Deterioration is shown by ↑ respiratory rate, ↓ pulse rate, BP ↑ initially and then ↓ (a pre-morbid sign).
- On discharge give verbal and written information of symptoms/signs to observe for and when to return.

MICRO-case

A 24-year-old male presents after being hit in the head with a cricket ball. The injury caused him to lose consciousness for 1 or 2 minutes (according to his friends) and he fell to the floor.

He has a headache that is relieved with co-codamol. On examination there is obvious bruising and bogginess where the ball hit him, but no obvious clinical fracture. His GCS is now 15/15 and has been since admission, and he wants to leave the department. He has not yet had a skull x-ray.

Three hours following self-discharge, he collapses. On readmission to the emergency department, one pupil is fixed and dilated and he is urgently transferred to the local neurosurgical unit.

Learning points:

- Remember that extradural haematomas often present following a lucid period.
- If in doubt admit and monitor GCS closely, especially if consciousness was lost.
- Consider imaging all patients with significant head injury.
- Collateral history from witness is invaluable in patients who lose consciousness.

General surgery

10.5 BURNS

10.5.1 DEFINITION

- Damage to skin and subcutaneous tissue in response to thermal, electrical, chemical, frictional, cold or radiation injury.
- By far the commonest type in the UK is a thermal burn, caused mostly by dry burn, e.g. flame, but can be from a wet burn, e.g. scalding.

10.5.2 ASSESSMENT OF EXTENT OF BURN

Size of burn

- The patient's palm is ~1% of his or her total body surface area (TBSA) and can be useful to determine extent of small or very large burns.
- Wallace's rule of 9's is useful in initial assessment (see Figure 10.2).
- It is important to use the appropriate chart for the patient's age.

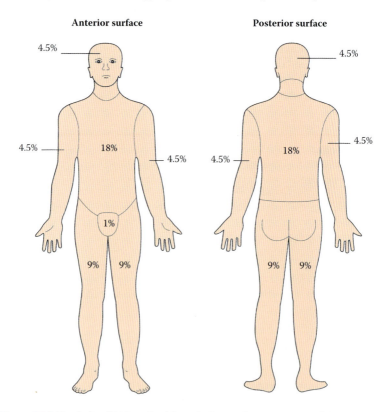

Anterior surface   **Posterior surface**

Figure 10.2 The 'rule of 9's' method for calculating the proportion of the total body surface area that has been burnt. (From: *Browse's Introduction to the Signs and Symptoms of Surgical Disease, 4th Edition*, Figure 3.20, p. 64.)

Depth of burn (see Table 10.2)

- Difficult to assess accurately since burns tend to be dynamic and evolve over time.
- Figures 10.3 and 10.4 show the characteristics of different burn depths.

Table 10.2 Difference between different depths of burns.

	SUPERFICIAL PARTIAL THICKNESS (FIGURE 10.3)	DEEP PARTIAL THICKNESS (FIGURE 10.4)	FULL THICKNESS
Layers involved	Epidermis and upper layers of dermis.	Epidermis and most of dermis.	Epidermis and dermis.
Colour	Pink.	Pink/red.	White/charred.
Blisters	Yes.	Yes.	No.
Capillary refill	Blanches and refills.	Non-blanching.	Non-blanching.
Pain	Yes.	Yes.	No.
Sensation	Normal.	Reduced.	Insensate.
Outcome	Heals well with no scar.	Heals slowly with scarring.	Unlikely to heal if large or heals slowly with severe scarring.

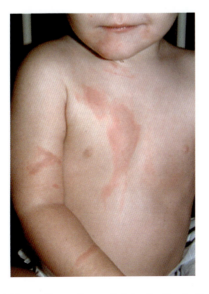

Figure 10.3 Superficial burn. (From: *Browse's Introduction to the Investigation and Management of Surgical Disease*, 4th Edition, Figure 5.19, p. 108.)

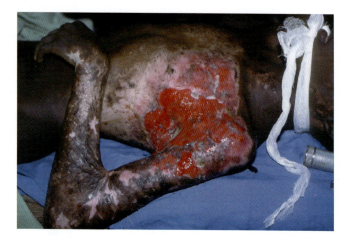

Figure 10.4 A mixture of partial-thickness and full-thickness burns. (From: *Browse's Introduction to the Signs and Symptoms of Surgical Disease, 4th Edition,* Figure 3.21, p. 65.)

10.5.3 INITIAL MANAGEMENT OF ACUTE BURN

- Like any emergency, management should take the ABC approach.

> **MICRO-facts**
>
> Signs of potential inhalation injury:
> - Burns on neck, around mouth, on palate or nasal passages.
> - Soot in oropharynx or nostrils.
> - Hoarse voice.
> - Hypoxia.
> - Carboxyhaemoglobin.
> - Stridor, tachypnoea and dyspnoea are late signs.

Airway and breathing

- If suspected smoke inhalation, early intubation is indicated to prevent airway obstruction and death.
- If severe airway obstruction, a tracheostomy may be needed.
- High-flow oxygen through non-rebreathing mask.
- Perform ABG and check carbon monoxide levels.

Fluid resuscitation

- Burn injuries lead to large inflammatory exudation of proteins and solutes into the extravascular space.
- This occurs within the first 6–12 hours post-injury (not post-arrival into the emergency department!) and starts to slow by 36 hours.

- Fluid loss is dependent on size of burn:
    - ≥15% total body surface area (TBSA) in adults and ≥10% in children will lead to circulatory shock.
- Insert a large-bore cannula and catheterise (to monitor output; keep urine output 0.5–1 mL/hour in adults, 1–2 mL/hour in children).
- Use the Parkland formula to calculate the fluid requirements (usually Hartmann's solution).
    - Give half in the first 8 hours (from the time of injury), and half in the next 16 hours.

MICRO-facts

Parkland formula:
Amount of fluid in ml = % TBSA × weight in kg × 4 ml.

Analgesia
- Cool wound with running water for 10 minutes.
- Temporary use of cling-film as dressing reduces evaporation and pain.
- If small burn, simple oral analgesia may be sufficient.
- If large burn, IV opiate analgesia will be needed (do not use IM route).

Nutrition
- Burn injuries lead to a highly catabolic state.
- If burns >20% TBSA, insert a nasogastric (NG) tube within 6 hours to prevent stress ulceration of the stomach (Curling's ulcers).

10.5.4 MANAGEMENT OF THE BURN WOUND
- Depends on burn depth (Figure 10.5).
- Assess if an escharotomy is needed:
    - An escharotomy is an incision along the full length of the burn to relieve compression due to oedema in circumferential full-thickness burns.
    - The incision is in the mid-axial line and extends down to the fascia.
    - Necessary if blood flow to a limb is occluded or respiratory movement restricted.
    - Escharotomies should be performed in an operating theatre by a burns specialist if at all possible.
- If assessment indicates that escharotomy may be required, discuss **urgently** with the local burns unit and arrange transfer.
- After escharotomy the principles of management are the same regardless of the size of the burn.

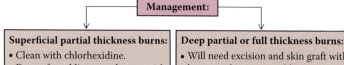

Superficial partial thickness burns:	Deep partial or full thickness burns:
• Clean with chlorhexidine. • De-roof any blisters and cover with paraffin impregnated gauze or a silicone sheet (e.g. Mepetil). • Change dressings twice weekly. • Will heal within 2 weeks.	• Will need excision and skin graft within 72 hours as skin is not viable. • If minor (<20% TBSA) it may be appropriate to delay grafting for a few days. • Physiotherapy is essential post-operatively to prevent contracture and maintain joint mobility.

Figure 10.5 General management plan for burns.

MICRO-facts

Indications for referral to specialist burn unit:

- Deep partial-thickness or full-thickness burn.
- Burns > 10% TBSA in adults, > 5% in children.
- Patient < 1 year or > 65 years old.
- Significant associated injury or medical comorbidity.
- Pregnant women.
- Burns involving face, hands, feet, genitalia, perineum or a joint.
- Circumferential burns (i.e. needing escharotomy).
- Suspected inhalation injury.
- Chemical or electrical burn.
- Suspected non-accidental injury.
- You should have a low threshold for discussing any patient who has sustained a burn injury with the nearest burn unit.

MICRO-case

A 32-year-old female presents to the emergency department with burns to her left arm and anterior torso an hour after her gas hob malfunctioned whilst she was cooking.

You follow the ABCDE approach. She is maintaining her own airway and there is no evidence of smoke inhalation injury. She is tachypnoeic with a RR of 18, but her chest sounds clear with equal air entry bilaterally. She is tachycardic with a HR of 105 and her BP is 105/70. You commence high-flow oxygen and insert a wide-bore IV line in her contra-lateral arm.

On examination she has painful dark pink/red burns with blisters that appear to be deep partial thickness. Using the 'rule of 9's' you estimate that she has suffered ~27% TSBA burns. She weighs 60 kg. Using the Parkland formula you calculate that she requires 6480 mL of IV fluid (additional to her daily maintenance fluid) over the first 24 hours.

continued...

You commence fluid resuscitation with Hartmann's solution (giving 3240 mL over the next 7 hours), apply running cold water to the affected areas and dress with cling-film before contacting the local burn unit.

Learning points:

- Adults with >10% TSBA burns need discussion with a burn unit.
- Large quantities of intravenous fluids may be required.
- Escharotomy may be needed in patients with circumferential burns to the limbs or thorax.

11 Post-operative care

11.1 POST-OPERATIVE CARE ON THE SURGICAL WARD

- Most post-operative surgical patients will recover quickly and uneventfully from their surgery.
  - Some, however, may be slow to progress or develop complications. It is important to review patients regularly and thoroughly so that these issues can be identified and addressed.
- Ward round notes should be documented legibly with the date and time.
  - They should include information about the patient's progress, and there must be a clear plan for the day.
  - This provides clear information about the current status of the patient should members of the on-call team be asked to review him or her.
- The following (where relevant) should be reviewed daily in every patient.

11.1.1 OBSERVATIONS

- Basic observations should be checked and recorded every day on a chart to allow trends to be identified.
- When patients become unwell on the wards, the observations have often shown evidence of deterioration in the preceding few hours. It is therefore important to monitor and act on any changes as they occur.
- Pulse, blood pressure (BP), respiratory rate, oxygen saturations and temperature should all be noted.
- Fluid balance (input vs. output) should also be charted and assessed.

11.1.2 PAIN MANAGEMENT

- Analgesia requirements will vary from patient to patient and will also depend on the type of surgery.
- Post-operatively patients may have an epidural or patient-controlled analgesia (PCA) that will need reviewing.
  - These methods are effective analgesics but prevent early mobilisation.
- The 'analgesia ladder' is a good method of prescribing analgesia in patients with acute pain (see Figure 11.1).

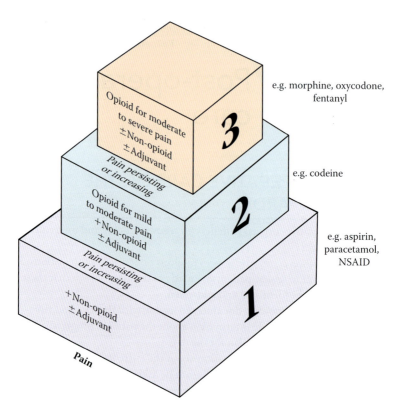

e.g. morphine, oxycodone, fentanyl

e.g. codeine

e.g. aspirin, paracetamol, NSAID

Figure 11.1 The analgesia ladder. (From: *Baker and Aldoori*, Figure 3.3, p. 25.)

- Remember that patients who are not tolerating oral analgesia will need alternative routes (e.g. PR, subcutaneous, IV).

11.1.3 NUTRITION

- With most surgical procedures, patients are reasonably well nourished pre-operatively and may begin eating and drinking on the same day post-operatively.
- There are certain circumstances, however, where supplementary nutrition may be required to prevent malnourishment and aid recovery. These include patients with:
  - malabsorption, chronic intestinal fistulae or high-output stomas;
  - intestinal obstruction or ileus;
  - chronic liver disease;
  - advanced neoplasia;
  - emergency patients who have had a period of starvation or poor oral intake due to nausea and vomiting.

General surgery

- Enteral feeding is the preferable route of supplemental nutrition if the gastrointestinal (GI) tract is functioning. There are several methods of increasing calorie intake, including:
  - oral supplements (e.g. Fortisips™);
  - fine-bore nasogastric (NG) feeding (e.g. overnight);
  - insertion of feeding jejunostomy (this may be inserted at the time of surgery, e.g. for patients having oesophagectomy).
- Parenteral feeding should be considered when nutrition cannot be supplemented through the GI tract.
  - Usually administered via a central vein to avoid the risk of phlebitis from the high osmolarity feed.
  - Complications of total parenteral nutrition (TPN) include:
    - sepsis or thrombosis (from the central line);
    - electrolyte imbalance (bloods should be monitored daily);
    - hyperglycaemia and liver damage (patients may require concurrent insulin infusion).

11.1.4 CATHETERS

- Urinary catheters may be inserted for monitoring purposes or to drain the bladder following urological procedures or where there is significant immobility post-operatively.
  - They are a potential source of sepsis and should be removed as early as is feasible.
  - Patients are monitored during a trial without catheter (TWOC) to ensure they are able to urinate following removal.
  - Check that there are no specific instructions regarding catheter removal (e.g. a patient who has had intra-operative bladder damage may require a cystogram prior to removal of the catheter).

11.1.5 NASOGASTRIC TUBES

- Nasogastric (NG) tubes are not routinely used but may be required in certain patients.
  - They may be used for post-operative nutrition (usually fine-bore).
  - They may be used to decompress the GI tract following GI surgery.
- NG output should be taken into account when calculating fluid balance.
- Patients with high NG aspirates need their electrolytes checking daily to ensure these are replaced.

11.1.6 DRAINS

- Drains are placed to prevent post-operative collections following surgery.
- They may also provide vital clues as to post-operative complications, e.g.:
  - Bile in a drain following a cholecystectomy suggests a leak and should prompt further investigation.

General surgery

- Large output of fresh blood indicates active bleeding and should trigger urgent action.

11.1.7 WOUNDS

- Wounds should be checked regularly to ensure healing and to look for evidence of infection.
- If there are skin sutures or clips, these should be reviewed for removal (usually 5–10 days post-operatively, depending on the site of the incision).

11.1.8 PRINCIPLES OF ENHANCED RECOVERY

- Surgery results in a stress response, and there several factors that impact on post-operative recovery (Figure 11.2).
- The enhanced recovery programme is a set of principles aimed at improving patient outcomes and speeding up patient's recovery after surgery (Figure 11.3).
- The four main elements involved are:
  - pre-operative assessment, pre-admission planning and preparation;
  - reducing the physical stress of the operation;
  - structured peri-operative and immediate post-operative management;
  - early mobilisation.

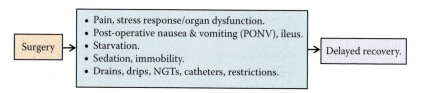

Figure 11.2 Surgical stresses.

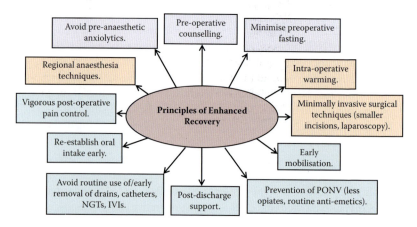

Figure 11.3 The principles of enhanced recovery.

11.2 GENERAL POST-OPERATIVE COMPLICATIONS

- It is important to remember that not all post-operative complications will present in the same way. When reviewing a patient who 'doesn't look right' following surgery, you must remember to take into account the following points:
    - any specific complaints (e.g. do they complain of abdominal pain or vomiting following an abdominal procedure?);
    - the surgery they have undergone;
    - how long ago they had their surgery;
    - their general appearance (e.g. do they appear pale or in pain?);
    - their recent observations and any obvious trends;
    - their most recent investigations.
        - If they have not had any, it may be appropriate to take appropriate bloods or request a chest x-ray (CXR), for example, depending on the examination findings.
- Try and follow a logical sequence whenever you are asked to review an unwell patient.
- Remember, if you are unsure what is going on, ask for senior help.

MICRO-facts

Classification:
- Primary haemorrhage:
    - Occurs at time of the operation.
- Reactionary haemorrhage:
    - Occurs within 24 hours of the operation.
    - Usually venous and caused by slipping of ligature or relaxation of vasospasm.
- Secondary haemorrhage:
    - Occurs at 7–14 days post-operatively.
    - Usually due to re-establishment of vessel patency secondary to infection or due to thrombus disintegration.
    - Haemorrhage may be fatal and heralded by a bright red 'warning' bleed.

11.2.1 HAEMORRHAGE

Clinical features

- Signs of shock.:
    - hypotension;
    - tachycardia;

- - low JVP;
  - pallor;
  - agitation/confusion.
- Swelling at wound site.
- Blood in drains or on wound dressing.

Management
- ABCDE approach.
  - Give high-flow oxygen.
  - Establish venous access with large-bore cannulae.
  - Commence fluid resuscitation with crystalloid fluid.
    - E.g. normal saline (0.9%).
  - Catheterise to monitor fluid resuscitation.
  - Apply compression to bleeding wound.
  - Check haemoglobin and clotting screen.
  - Obtain urgent cross-match in case a blood transfusion is required.
- If bleeding doesn't stop with pressure or the patient is haemodynamically unstable, then urgent re-operation may be indicated to control the source.

11.2.2 SEPSIS AND THE SYSTEMIC INFLAMMATORY RESPONSE SYNDROME (SIRS)

- **Sepsis** = SIRS in the presence of infection proven by organism culture.
- **MODS** = multiple organ dysfunction syndrome as a result of SIRS.
  - Patient requires interventions to maintain normal homeostasis.
- Pathophysiology of sepsis: See Figure 11.4.
- Loss of homeostasis of normal acute phase inflammatory response due to presence of greater titres of pro-inflammatory cytokines than anti-inflammatory cytokines (Figure 11.5).

MICRO-facts
For diagnosis of SIRS ≥ 2 the following should be present:
- Temp > 38°C or < 36°C.
- HR > 90 bpm.
- RR > 20 breaths/minute or $PaCO_2$ < 4.3 kPa.
- WBC > 12×10^9/L or < 4×10^9/L.

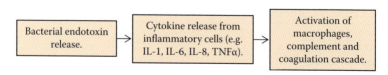

Figure 11.4 The pathophysiology of sepsis.

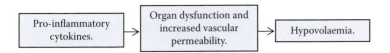

Figure 11.5 How sepsis results in hypovolaemia.

- 'Septic screen' investigations to determine the underlying cause:
  - Full systematic examination.
    - Remember to look at surgical wounds.
  - Blood cultures.

> **MICRO-facts**
>
> ABG may show ↓ $PaCO_2$ and a metabolic acidosis (i.e. ↓ pH and ↓ HCO_3^-).

- Stool MC&S if there is diarrhoea.
  - Urine dip and MC&S to identify any urinary tract infection (UTI).
  - CXR to identify any lower respiratory tract infection.
- Other investigations may help elicit the extent of organ dysfunction:
  - Full blood count (FBC), urea and electrolytes (U&E), liver function tests (LFTs), clotting screen;
  - ABG;
  - ECG.

Management
- Urgent treatment is necessary to prevent further organ damage.
- May need intensive treatment unit (ITU) care for organ support.
- Airway and breathing:
  - Give high-flow oxygen if dyspnoeic.
- Circulation:
  - IV crystalloid fluids if hypotensive via large-bore cannula.
- Empirical antibiotic cover until results of septic screen are known, then tailor antibiotics to organism.
- Close monitoring of vital observations and blood results for signs of improvement or deterioration.

11.2.3 WOUND INFECTION

Aetiology
- Skin organisms, e.g. *Staphylococcus aureus*.
- Contamination from surgical opening of viscera, especially bowel, biliary tree or urinary tract.
- Contamination from staff in operating theatre, e.g. poor scrubbing technique or nasal/skin carriage of *Staphylococci*.

- Surgery involving poorly vascularised tissue.
- Patient factors, e.g. diabetes mellitus, immunosuppression, malnutrition, arteriopathy, smoking.

Clinical features

- Usually develops a few days post-operatively.
- Signs of inflammation will be present, i.e.:
    - erythema;
    - warmth;
    - swelling;
    - pain;
    - malaise;
    - pyrexia.
- Pus discharging from wound.
- Tachycardia.

Investigations

- Swab wound for MC&S.
- FBC shows ↑ white cell count (WCC) secondary to infection.
- Blood cultures.

Management

- Clean and dress the wound adequately.
- Drain any pus collections.
- Empirical use of antibiotics to cover likely organisms (e.g. flucloxacillin if *Staphylococci*) until results of septic screen are known.
- If fulminant sepsis see Section 11.2.2.
- If concerned about methicillin-resistant *Staphylococcus aureus* (MRSA) as causative agent consult microbiology.

> ### MICRO-facts
>
> Subcutaneous abscess management:
> - Usually occurs 5–10 days post-operatively.
> - Will need incision, washout and drainage.
> - Wound is usually left open to heal by secondary intent with granulation tissue.

11.2.4 PARALYTIC ILEUS

- This is where there is cessation of normal peristaltic movement in the bowel.
- Most commonly follows abdominal surgery where the bowel has been handled.
    - May also be due to an anastomotic leak or intra-abdominal abscess, and this should always be considered.
    - May be mistaken for obstruction, or vice versa (Figure 11.6).

Ileus vs. obstruction in the post-operative patient

Ileus:	Obstruction:
• Abdominal distension, often tense and hyperresonant. • Absolute constipation. • Vomiting, high NG aspirates. • Absent bowel sounds. • Abdominal pain is usually absent. • AXR may show gaseous distension throughout.	• Consider if persists longer than 4 days – further imaging (e.g. CT scan) may be indicated. • Bowel sounds high pitched, 'tinkling'. • Abdominal pain (usually colicky). • AXR usually shows dilated loops of bowel and may show a 'cut-off' with no gas below the obstruction. • Obstruction may occur in the immediate post-op period due to adhesions.

Figure 11.6 Differences between ileus and obstruction.

- Other causes include metabolic disturbance and drugs (anti-cholingergics).
- Ileus also occurs in patients admitted to ITU or surviving major trauma.
- Management.
    - Patients will need IV fluid (with electrolytes) to maintain hydration and NG tube placing if vomiting and distension.
    - Patients may require parenteral feeding if persistent to avoid malnourishment.
    - Monitor electrolytes, especially as some electrolyte imbalances may precipitate paralytic ileus.
    - There may be large accumulation of fluid within the gut and needs to be accounted for in fluid management.
        - Invasive monitoring is often needed to ensure patient is not fluid depleted/overloaded.

11.2.5 PULMONARY ATELECTASIS

Definition
- Partial collapse of the lung due to alveolar collapse.
- Occurs when there is blockage of the small airways (commonly by mucus), leading to collapse distal to the obstruction, where superadded infection may occur.

Aetiology
- More common in smokers/chronic obstructive pulmonary disease (COPD) sufferers.
- Post-operative pain (abdominal or thoracic surgery) and opioid analgesia overuse lead to shallow inspiration and inhibition of coughing.

General surgery

Clinical features

- Mild collapse in a fit and healthy patient may not be symptomatic, or may cause only mild pyrexia.
- More severe obstruction and collapse may lead to consolidation with dyspnoea and tachypnoea.
- On auscultation there may be reduced air entry, bronchial breathing and dullness to percussion.
  - There may also be an associated drop in oxygen saturations.

Investigation

- CXR will demonstrate opacified lung tissue and rarely mediastinal shift due to expansion of other lobes.
- ABG to assess for hypoxia and hypercapnia.
- Sputum should be sent for culture.
- Differentiation from LRTI:
  - No raised white cell count in atelectasis.
  - Productive cough and purulent sputum in infection.
  - Consolidation on chest x-ray.

Management

- Chest physiotherapy may be useful pre- and post-operatively.
- Adequate analgesia to allow deep breathing and coughing.
- Nebulised bronchodilators may aid coughing of secretions.
- In severe cases, bronchoscopy may be indicated to remove mucus plugs and the most severe may require intubation and mechanical ventilation.

11.2.6 ACUTE RESPIRATORY DISTRESS SYNDROME (ARDS)

- Respiratory distress with reduced lung compliance and characteristic CXR changes (diffuse lung opacification). There are abnormalities on ABG with $\downarrow$ PaO_2 but $\leftrightarrow PaCO_2$, regardless of positive end expiratory pressure.

Aetiology

- Pulmonary causes:
  - pneumonia;
  - inhalation of smoke/vomit/water/corrosives;
  - embolism;
  - lung contusion.
- Non-pulmonary causes:
  - sepsis/SIRS [e.g. pancreatitis, disseminated intravascular coagulation (DIC)];
  - massive transfusion;
  - severe allergy;
  - head injury.

Clinical features

- Unexplained tachypnoea, dyspnoea, increasing hypoxaemia, cyanosis.
- On auscultation fine crepitations are heard throughout the lungs.

Investigation

- CXR shows a 'whiteout' with costophrenic angle sparing.
- ABG shows resistant hypoxia with normal CO_2 (until late in the disease).
  - Differential diagnoses include pulmonary oedema (in ARDS there will no cardiomegaly and no response to furosemide) and pneumonia.

Management

- Admit to high-dependency unit (HDU)/ITU for mechanical ventilation.
- Treat any underlying conditions (e.g. sepsis).
- Monitor the fluid balance, central venous pressure, and look for secondary lung infection and renal failure.

Prognosis

- Depends on the aetiology (pulmonary causes generally better), age of the patient and presence of more than one organ failure.
- The mortality has improved but still remains at around 30–40%.

MICRO-print

Pathophysiology of ARDS:
- Increased pulmonary vascular permeability and interstitial oedema with type 1 pneumocyte damage.
  - Reduced alveolar surface area and ventilation-perfusion mismatch.
- Constriction of pulmonary vasculature to shunt blood.
  - Pulmonary hypertension.
- Fibroblasts attempt to repair damage lung resulting in fibrosis.

11.2.7 ACUTE KIDNEY INJURY (AKI)

- A rapid reduction in renal function with an inability to maintain electrolyte balance, acid-base homeostasis and urine production.

MICRO-facts

AKI is defined when one of the following criteria is met:
- Rise in serum creatinine of ≥26 μmol/L within 48 hours.
- Rise in serum creatinine by ≥1.5-fold from the patient's normal level.
- Urine output of <0.5 mL/kg/hour for >6 consecutive hours.

General surgery

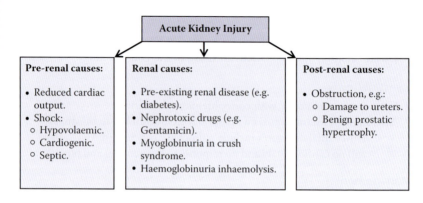

Figure 11.7 Causes of AKI.

Aetiology

- May be divided into pre-renal, renal and post-renal causes (Figure 11.7).
- In the post-op patient by far the commonest cause is dehydration, i.e. pre-renal.

Investigations

- U&E to monitor creatinine and to check for hyperkalaemia.
- ABG may show acidosis.

> **MICRO-facts**
>
> **Normal urine output:** Around 1500–2000 mL/day (or >1 mL/kg/hour).
> **Oliguria:** 100–400 mL/day (or <0.3 mL/kg/hour).
> **Anuria:** Anything <100 mL/day.

- ECG if potassium is raised.
- Urinalysis.
- Renal tract ultrasound scan (USS) if obstruction is suspected.

Management

- Insert a urinary catheter if not already catheterised and monitor output.
  - Check catheter is not blocked.
  - Examine abdomen for signs of distended bladder.
- Intravenous fluid challenge and check for response.
- Stop any nephrotoxic drugs.
- Do not give furosemide, as this may further dehydrate the patient.

11.2.8 VENOUS THROMBOEMBOLISM (VTE): DVT/PE

> **MICRO-facts**
>
> Predisposing factors for VTE:
> - Trauma.
> - Lower limb or pelvic surgery.
> - Malignancy.
> - Figure 11

- Clot formation in the venous system, composed mostly of fibrinogen deposits.
  - These may form in the deep arm or leg veins.
  - May release emboli, which can lodge in the lungs, causing a pulmonary embolism (PE).

Aetiology
- Caused by a collections of factors, known as Virchow's triad (see Figure 11.8).

Clinical features
- Usually develop symptoms over 7 days post-op.
- See Table 11.1.

Investigations
- D-dimer blood test—if this is normal it excludes venous thromboembolism.
- Doppler ultrasound to assess venous flow in the limb.

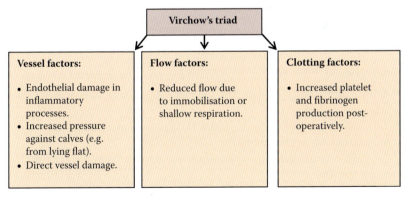

Figure 11.8 Virchow's triad.

General surgery

Table 11.1 Signs and symptoms of VTE.

	DVT	PE

Symptoms	• Calf pain.
	• Stiffness.
	• Fever.
		• Sudden onset of:
		  – Dyspnoea.
		  – Pleuritic chest pain.
		  – Haemoptysis.

Signs	• Unilateral leg swelling (usually lower leg but may be whole leg in pelvic thrombosis).
	• Calf tenderness.
	• Warm skin.
	• Dilatation of superficial veins.
		• Cardiovascular instability (hypotension, tachycardia, peripheral vasoconstriction).
		• Pleural rub.
		• Rarely coarse crackles over affected lung.
		• In a large PE there may be:
		  – Cardiovascular collapse.
		  – Raised JVP.
		  – Right heart heave.
		  – Wide split second heart sound.

- CXR may show linear atelectasis, costophrenic angle blunting, wedge-shaped pulmonary infarct (rare to see) in PE.
- ECG changes (classically, but rarely, S1, Q3, T3 demonstrating evidence of right heart strain) in PE.
  - S wave in lead I, Q wave and inverted T wave in lead III.
  - More commonly shows only a sinus tachycardia.
- ABG may show hypoxia.
- Computed tomography pulmonary angiography (CTPA) is the gold standard investigation for diagnosis of a PE.

Management

- Immediate resuscitation with ABCDE method, give high-flow oxygen and adequate analgesia.
- Low molecular weight heparin (LMWH) is given to prevent further propagation of the clot and further clot formation.
  - Convert to oral anticoagulation after 5 days and continue for 3–6 months.
- Patients awaiting surgery at high risk of PE (e.g. a cancer patient with a new deep vein thrombosis (DVT)) may require an IVC filter to enable them to undergo their operation without anticoagulation whilst preventing embolism.

Part II

Self-assessment

12

Pre-operative care

12.1 PRE-OPERATIVE CARE EMQs

1. For each of the following clinical scenarios, please choose the single **most** useful pre-operative test you would perform. Each answer may be used once, more than once or not at all.

Blood glucose	Echocardiography
Clotting screen	LFTs
Cross-match	Pulmonary function tests
CXR	Sickle cell test
ECG	Urinalysis

a. A 27-year-old Afro-Caribbean patient who is fit and well and scheduled to undergo an elective inguinal hernia repair.

b. A slim, fit and well 25-year-old female due to undergo excision of a fibroadenoma and is found to have a new, asymptomatic, mitral regurgitant heart murmur on examination.

c. An otherwise fit and well 29-year-old female who is undergoing total thyroidectomy for a large goitre and is clinically and biochemically euthyroid.

12.2 PRE-OPERATIVE CARE EMQ ANSWERS

1. a. Answer: Sickle cell test.

   A sickle cell test should be performed in patients with a family history of sickle cell disease and considered in all African or Caribbean patients undergoing surgery. This patient is otherwise American Society of Anasthesiologists (ASA 1), undergoing a simple procedure, and so would routinely not need any other pre-operative tests.

   b. Answer: Echocardiography.

   This woman is again ASA 1, undergoing a simple procedure. However a new murmur mandates investigation, the most appropriate of which is an echo, as it will provide you with the most information. It is most likely to be 'floppy mitral valve syndrome', which is usually a non-haemodynamically significant murmur often seen in slim young females.

c. Answer: Chest x-ray.

Again ASA 1, as she is euthyroid. However she is having surgery for a goitre, which may be causing tracheal deviation. This will be demonstrated on a plain CXR.

12.3 PRE-OPERATIVE CARE SBAs

For each of the questions below, select the single best answer. Each option may be used once only.

1. A patient is referred via the 2-week wait system with bright red rectal bleeding and a possible rectal mass. He undergoes flexible sigmoidoscopy and is found to have an annular, constricting cancer of the recto-sigmoid that the endoscopist was unable to pass—there is a concern that the patient may soon obstruct. Biopsies confirm adenocarcinoma. The patient undergoes staging tests and is booked for a high anterior resection. What is the NCEPOD classification for this patient?
   a. Elective.
   b. Emergency.
   c. Scheduled.
   d. Soon.
   e. Urgent.

2. You pre-assess a 70-year-old man who is listed for an inguinal hernia repair under general anaesthetic. Which of the following would cause you or your anaesthetist to cancel the operation?
   a. Aortic valve area of 0.83 cm^2 on a recent echocardiogram.
   b. LV-aortic gradient of 19 mmHg on a recent echocardiogram.
   c. Patient who is on warfarin for atrial fibrillation.
   d. Patient with left bundle branch block (LBBB) on his ECG since a heart attack 2 years ago.
   e. Recent aortic valve replacement surgery.

3. A 53-year-old man with ischaemic heart disease is due to undergo an elective hernia repair. He suffers with angina and has to use his GTN spray when he climbs a flight of stairs or a steep incline. He lives alone in a bungalow. What ASA grade would he fall into?
   a. ASA 1.
   b. ASA 2.
   c. ASA 3.
   d. ASA 4.
   e. ASA 5.

12.4 PRE-OPERATIVE CARE SBA ANSWERS

1. Answer: Scheduled.

   This patient is placed on the waiting list but surgery should be performed in 4 weeks, as the patient has a malignancy, under the present UK government cancer waiting times guidelines. If he were to obstruct completely, surgery may become more urgent and need to be performed as 'urgent'. 'Soon' is not part of the NCEPOD classification.

2. Answer: Aortic valve area of 0.83 cm^2.

   A valve area of less than 1 cm^2 is classified as severe aortic stenosis. This patient needs to be referred to the cardiothoracic surgeons for a valve replacement before undergoing any elective surgery. An LV-aortic gradient of 19 mmHg is normal. A patient on warfarin for AF needs his warfarin stopped 5 days prior to his operation to normalise his INR, but the operation can still go ahead. This patient had his heart attack more than 6 months ago and so should be okay to undergo a general anaesthetic. A patient who has recently undergone aortic valve surgery should be fit enough for hernia surgery but may be on anti-coagulants that will need heparin or LMWH cover during the peri-operative period.

3. Answer: ASA 3.

   This man's ischaemic heart disease limits normal activity (i.e. climbing a flight of stairs); however he is not incapacitated by it and manages to live independently.

13 Lumps and bumps

13.1 LUMPS AND BUMPS EMQs

1. For each of the following clinical scenarios please choose the most appropriate diagnosis. Each answer may be used once, more than once or not at all.

   Abscess   Lipoma
   Liposarcoma   Neurofibroma
   Umbilical hernia   Paraumbilical hernia
   Epigastric hernia   Sebaceous cyst
   Femoral hernia   Spigelian hernia

   a. A 37-year-old female presents to her GP with a 2-week history of a lump immediately below her umbilicus. The lump is causing slight discomfort. On examination there is a 3 cm mobile, midline subcutaneous swelling, which is non-tender. It does not transilluminate and is reducible. Bowel sounds can be heard on auscultation.

   b. A 30-year-old man presents to you with a non-tender, 3-cm spherical lump on the side of his torso in the right lower abdomen. It has been present for over 5 years and is not enlarging. It is soft, mobile, of normal colour, not warm to touch and non-adherent to the underlying tissue. You are able to move the skin over the lump and the lump over the abdominal wall. There is no cough impulse and it is non-reducible.

   c. A 75-year-old female presents to her GP with a lump that has developed over the past week in the left groin. It is tender to touch. On inspection there is a 3-cm tender mass in the left medial groin, just below and lateral to the pubic tubercle. There is associated mild erythema but the patient is apyrexial. The mass is non-reducible and does not transilluminate.

2. For each of the following clinical scenarios please choose the most appropriate diagnosis. Each answer may be used once, more than once or not at all.

   Angiosarcoma   Hidradinitis suppurativa
   Basal cell carcinoma   Kaposi's sarcoma
   Benign pigmented naevus   Malignant melanoma
   Infected sebaceous cyst   Haematoma
   Haemangioma   Squamous cell carcinoma

a. A 45-year-old male presents with a 3-month history of an area of raised red skin in his underarm area. The area is tender. On examination he has a papular rash with erythema. There are several 'heads' with pustules. His contralateral axilla has a similar but milder appearance.

b. A 71-year-old female presents with a bruised appearance on her left breast, which has been present for 3 months and is growing. She can recall no history of preceding trauma and is concerned that it is not fading with time. She is fit and well with no other health problems. She has a past history of left breast cancer that was treated by wide local excision and radiotherapy 9 years ago.

c. You a requested by a GP to see a 67-year-old male in your general clinic under the '2-week wait' service. He presented with a lump on his back, which his wife had noticed had been there for several years, but now it seems to be growing. On inspecting this lump you see that he has a 1.5 cm lesion, which has a mix of light and dark pigmentation, with a poorly defined border. The skin around it is excoriated. The lesion itches, and has left blood on his shirt a few times, but he thinks this is where he caught it itching. What is the most likely diagnosis?

13.2 LUMPS AND BUMPS EMQ ANSWERS

1. a. Answer: Paraumbilical hernia.
   The key is the location and the reducibility. Umbilical hernias are only seen in babies and children.

   b. Answer: Lipoma.
   This is a common location for lipomata, which are soft and mobile—key features of this lump. They are also slow-growing and often have been present for many years.

   c. Answer: Femoral hernia.
   The location in relation to the pubic tubercle, as well as the patient's age, helps elicit this diagnosis. In the case described, the hernia is incarcerated and becoming strangulated (the fact that it is irreducible denotes incarceration, and the fact that it is tender denotes strangulation or ischaemia of the hernia sac contents.

2. a. Hidradanitis supprativa.
   The description sounds like the patient may have several abscesses—a common misdiagnosis for patients with hidradanitis supprativa. The diagnosis is confirmed by examining the contralateral axilla and finding a similar appearance.

   b. Answer: Angiosarcoma.

This is a common presentation of a radiation-induced angiosarcoma, following WLE of a breast lump with radiotherapy. The appearance and location are typical. Haemangioma may give a similar appearance but would have been present from birth or a younger age. Haematoma could be considered if the patient had only recently undergone WLE.

c. Answer: Malignant melanoma.

This lesion has arisen in a pre-existing mole that has changed—the features of this new lesion are very suspicious of a malignant melanoma: itching, bleeding, irregular border and varying pigmentation.

13.3 LUMPS AND BUMPS SBAs

For each of the questions below, select the single best answer. Each option may be used once only.

1. Which of the following is not a sign of a malignant change in a pre-existing naevus?
   a. Erythema.
   b. Increase in size.
   c. Pain.
   d. Pruritis.
   e. Ulceration.

2. Which of the following organisms is most commonly associated with hidradinitis suppurativa?
   a. *Staphylococcus aureus.*
   b. *Staphylococcus epidermidis.*
   c. *Streptococcus pneumonia.*
   d. *Streptococcus pyogenes.*
   e. *Escherichia coli.*

3. Which of the following is **not** a common site for sebaceous cysts?
   a. Abdomen.
   b. Back.
   c. Scalp.
   d. Scrotum.
   e. Vulva.

13.4 LUMPS AND BUMPS SBA ANSWERS

1. Answer: Erythema.
   Although ulceration and bleeding of a mole are suspicious signs to look out for, erythema alone is not worrying. The other answers are all signs of possible malignant change.

2. Answer: *Staphylococcus aureus*.
   Staphylococcus aureus is the most common bacteria associated with infection of the apocrine sweat glands—hidradinitis supprativa. This species of bacteria commonly causes pus formation, or 'suppuration'. Rarely coliforms, such as *E. coli*, may be the causative organism.
3. Answer: Abdomen.
   The common sites for sebaceous cyst formation are scalp, face, neck, back, scrotum and vulva.

14.1 BREAST EMQs

1. For each of the following clinical scenarios please choose the most appropriate diagnosis. Each answer may be used once, more than once or not at all.

Benign breast change	Hidradinitis supprativa
Breast abscess	Inflammatory breast cancer
Breast cyst	Locally advanced breast cancer
Ductal carcinoma in situ	Lymph node
Fibroadenoma	Metastatic breast cancer

a. A 26-year-old female presents to her GP having noticed a discrete lump in the upper outer quadrant of her right breast 3 days previously. She is very worried about it, as both her mother and maternal aunt have had breast cancer in the past, aged 40 and 42, respectively. She says that it is painful when she touches it, though admits that this might be secondary to the number of times that she has examined it herself. There is no history of any recent trauma to the breast. On examination the lump is roughly 1 cm in size, is smooth and firm to touch and is fairly mobile within the breast. There are no other changes in either breast or axillae. What is the most likely diagnosis?

b. An 89-year-old female presents with a weeping sore on her left breast. She lives alone and has had problems with this for nearly a year but 'didn't want to bother anyone with it'. She is systemically well; however recently it has started bleeding through her clothes. On further examination she has a 4-cm mass with overlying skin ulceration. Axillary examination reveals palpable firm lymphadenopathy.

c. A 60-year-old female presents for breast screening and is recalled for further assessment of a 2-cm focus of linear, branching microcalcification in the breast. She has no symptoms and breast examination is completely normal.

14.2 BREAST EMQ ANSWERS

1. a. Answer: Fibroadenoma.

   Fibroadenomas are fairly common in this age group, and although this woman has a positive family history of breast cancer, she is unlikely to develop cancer at this point in her life. The features of this lump are also suggestive of a fibroadenoma.

   b. Answer: Locally advanced breast cancer.

   This woman has a fungating breast cancer that has eroded through the skin. The lymphadenopathy is almost certainly due to regional spread. The main differential would be a breast abscess; however you would expect the history to be very short and that the mass be associated with pain. Breast abscess is also very uncommon in this age group.

   c. Answer: Ductal carcinoma *in situ* (DCIS).

   This woman has DCIS; the linear pattern of the microcalcification outlines the abnormality tracking along the duct. She will be recalled for further mammographic and USS assessment, in conjunction with a biopsy of the abnormal area.

14.3 BREAST SBAs

For each of the questions below, select the single best answer. Each option may be used once only.

1. Which of the following is **not** an aetiological risk factor for breast cancer?
   a. Late first pregnancy.
   b. Late menarche.
   c. Late menopause.
   d. Low parity.
   e. Use of hormone replacement therapy.

14.4 BREAST SBA ANSWERS

1. Answer: Late menarche.

   Increased cumulative oestrogen exposure is thought to be an aetiological risk factor for the development of breast cancer; therefore early menarche would be a factor.

15 Endocrine

15.1 ENDOCRINE EMQs

1. For each of the following clinical scenarios please choose the most appropriate diagnosis. Each answer may be used once, more than once or not at all.

   Addison's disease   Hypothyroidism
   Conn's syndrome   Phaeochromocytoma
   Cushing's syndrome   Primary hyperparathyroidism
   Functional psychosis   Secondary hyperparathyroidism
   Hyperthyroidism   Tertiary hyperparathyroidism

   a. A 40-year-old female presents to her GP with the sensation of 'fluttering in her chest'. On further questioning it is noted that she has recently been losing weight and been having problems with feeling sweaty a lot of the time. She has also noticed that her periods have become closer together and heavier.

   b. A 32-year-old male presented to his GP with a new onset of headaches over a matter of weeks; they could come at any time of the day, and weren't associated with bending or coughing. He found he had been feeling increasingly anxious despite no new worries at work or at home.

   c. A 30-year-old female is being investigated for a history of recurrent renal stones, with associated background abdominal pain, and low mood. She has been increasingly thirsty but glucose tolerance testing is normal, and she has noticed she is generally weak and tired. Her renal function is normal.

2. For each of the following clinical scenarios please choose the most appropriate diagnosis. Each answer may be used once, more than once or not at all.

   Atrial fibrillation   Hyperthyroidism
   Cushing's disease   Hypothyroidism
   Conn's syndrome   MEN type 2A
   Diabetes mellitus   MEN type 2B
   Depression   Phaeochromocytoma

   a. An 18-year-old male plumber presents with numerous episodes of palpitations as well as a number of panic attacks that he describes as feeling 'as if the world is going to end'. He says that the episodes are often brought on at work when he is leaning into a bathtub or there is pressure on his abdomen. Examination appears normal except for a scar on his neck from previous surgery, arachnodactyly and tall stature. He states that he was adopted as a child.

b. A 35-year-old woman with a past medical history of highly active systemic lupus erythematosus presents to you with weight gain, polydipsia, polyuria and muscle weakness. On examination you notice a number of purple lines on her abdomen.

c. A 56-year-old woman with coeliac disease presents to you with a 6-month history of weight gain, tiredness, lethargy and difficulty concentrating at work. She mentions that her hair has recently been much drier than usual and she has started having to use a skin moisturiser on a daily basis.

15.2 ENDOCRINE EMQ ANSWERS

1. a. Answer: Hyperthyroidism.
   Both hyperthyroidism and phaeochromocytoma may cause palpitations; however the associated symptoms are more suggestive of a thyroid problem. You might expect headache or uncontrollable blood pressure if the diagnosis were phaeochromocytoma. You should examine the patient for the presence of a goitre and thyroid eye signs.

   b. Answer: Phaeochromocytoma.
   A phaeochromocytoma will raise the blood pressure, and this can cause headaches. These headaches are distinguished from those of raised intracranial pressure by being unaffected by bending and coughing (actions that further increase intracranial pressure). In patients diagnosed with phaeochromocytoma, it is important to exclude MEN syndromes.

   c. Answer: Primary hyperparathyroidism.
   The history described is that of stones, abdominal groans and psychic moans, pointing toward a diagnosis of hyperparathyroidism. As her renal function is normal, the most likely diagnosis is primary hyperparathyroidism.

2. a. Answer: MEN type 2B.
   This man has a typical presentation of a phaeochromocytoma, and although he has no positive family history of MEN, he was adopted as a child. The previous neck surgery and marfinoid appearance suggest an underlying genetic mutation in the form of MEN type 2B.

b. Answer: Cushing's disease.

This woman has a long history of SLE, which is likely to indicate long-term use of steroids. She has several typical manifestations of Cushing's disease, which in her case is causing impaired glucose tolerance or diabetes mellitus.

c. Answer: Hypothyroidism.

This woman is presenting with a few very common signs and symptoms of hypothyroidism. This disorder can be seen in patients with other autoimmune disorders, such as coeliac disease.

15.3 ENDOCRINE SBAs

For each of the questions below, select the single best answer. Each option may be used once only.

1. Which type of thyroid cancer displays 'Orphan Annie' nuclei on histopathological examination of the specimen?
   a. Anaplastic.
   b. Follicular.
   c. Lymphoma.
   d. Medullary.
   e. Papillary.
2. The following tumours are features of MEN type 1, **except** which?
   a. Adrenocortical.
   b. Gastrinoma.
   c. Medullary thyroid carcinoma.
   d. Parathyroid.
   e. Prolactinoma.

15.4 ENDOCRINE SBA ANSWERS

1. Answer: Papillary carcinoma.

   The histology of papillary carcinoma is that of pale nuclei, described as 'Orphan Annie' nuclei—their presence is diagnostic of this type of thyroid cancer.
2. Answer: Medullary thyroid carcinoma.

   This is a feature of both MEN type 2A and MEN type 2B but is not a feature of MEN type 1.

Self-assessment

16 Hepatobiliary

16.1 HEPATOBILIARY EMQs

1. For each of the following clinical scenarios please choose the most appropriate diagnosis. Each answer may be used once, more than once or not at all.

   Benign gallbladder polyp   Fibrolamellar carcinoma
   Carcinoma of the gallbladder   Hepatic adenoma
   Carcinoma head of pancreas   Hepatocellular carcinoma
   Carcinoma body of pancreas   Liver metastases
   Cholangiocarcinoma   Primary sclerosing cholangitis

   a. You see a 74-year-old female with a long history of symptomatic gallstones, who has previously refused surgery. She presents with persistent right upper quadrant pain, vomiting and nausea. There is associated unintentional weight loss of nearly a stone in the past 2 months. Her past medical history includes ulcerative colitis. What is the most likely diagnosis?

   b. A 44-year-old female presents with upper abdominal pain. She has not required any analgesia and her only medication is the oral contraceptive pill (OCP), which she has taken for 20 years. An ultrasound scan (USS) demonstrates a normal gallbladder, but demonstrates an incidental mass in the liver. What is this incidental finding?

   c. A 67-year-old male presents to his GP after a friend reported that his suntan looked 'rather yellow'. He denies any other symptoms, but on further questioning he has recently bought some new clothes that seemed too big and he has been feeling 'run down' for a few weeks. His only past medical history is that of type 1 diabetes mellitus. On examination he is jaundiced and you can palpate a central abdominal mass. Which is the most likely diagnosis?

2. For each of the following clinical scenarios please choose the most appropriate diagnosis. Each answer may be used once, more than once or not at all.

   Acute pancreatitis   Hepatitis
   Biliary colic   Myocardial infarction
   Cholangitis   Pancreatic malignancy
   Cholecystitis   Peptic ulcer
   Chronic pancreatitis   Pneumonia

a. A 42-year-old female presents to the emergency department with constant right upper quadrant pain for the past 24 hours. She has had previous episodes of similar pain that tend to come on after eating fatty foods but usually only last a few hours. She is nauseated and is tender in the right upper quadrant with a positive Murphy's sign. Her LFTs are normal. Her temperature is 38.4°C and her neutrophil count is elevated.

b. A 70-year-old female is admitted to the emergency department resus room with collapse. She is tachycardic, pyrexial and hypotensive. Clinically she is jaundiced with tenderness in the RUQ. Her WCC is 25×10^9 and her bilirubin is 230 mmol/L.

c. A 54-year-old male presents with upper abdominal pain that radiates through to the back and is associated with vomiting. He has a past medical history of insulin-dependent diabetes mellitus, and his regular medications include Creon™. He has had similar attacks in the past with multiple hospital attendances. His amylase is 50 iU.

16.2 HEPATOBILIARY EMQ ANSWERS

1. a. Answer: Carcinoma of the gallbladder.
   This history is similar to one of chronic cholecystitis, but when coupled with a recent history of weight loss in an elderly person with a long history of gallstone disease, cancer should be considered. There is an association with ulcerative colitis.

   b. Answer: Hepatic adenoma.
   In a person this young, cancer of the hepatobiliary system is unlikely, although not impossible. She has been taking the OCP for a long time, and this is associated with hepatic adenoma. They are commonly picked up as an incidental finding on imaging for other pathologies.

   c. Answer: Carcinoma head of pancreas.
   This history of painless, progressive jaundice with a central abdominal mass, weight loss and tiredness is typical of head of pancreas carcinoma and should prompt further investigation with CT scanning.

2. a. Answer: Cholecystitis.
   A positive Murphy's sign indicates gallbladder inflammation. The preceding history is suggestive of biliary colic that has now developed into cholecystitis.

   b. Answer: Cholangitis.
   This patient presents with the classical Charcot's triad: RUQ pain, fever and jaundice. She requires an ABCDE approach with aggressive fluid resuscitation and immediate administration of IV antibiotics. Definitive management will include identifying and relieving the biliary obstruction.

c. Answer: Chronic pancreatitis.

This man has a history of multiple attacks of pancreatitis secondary to alcohol excess. He is an insulin-dependent diabetic and is on enzyme replacement therapy, indicating that his pancreas no longer functions. The clinical syndrome with a normal amylase is typical of chronic pancreatitis.

16.3 HEPATOBILIARY SBAs

For each of the questions below, select the single best answer. Each option may be used once only.

1. Which of the following hormones is secreted by δ cells in the pancreas?
   a. Amylase.
   b. Glucagon.
   c. Insulin.
   d. Pancreatic polypeptide.
   e. Somatostatin.

2. Which of the following would cause you to score 1 on the Imrie scoring system?
   a. Albumin 30 g/L.
   b. Calcium 2.1 mmol/L.
   c. LDH 540 iU/L.
   d. PaO_2 9.1 kPa.
   e. Serum urea 15.2 mmol/L.

16.4 HEPATOBILIARY SBA ANSWERS

1. Answer: Somatostatin.

   Glucagon is secreted by α cells, insulin is secreted by β cells and pancreatic polypeptide is secreted by PP cells. Amylase is an enzyme, not a hormone, and is secreted by the exocrine pancreas.

2. Answer: Albumin 30 g/L.

   Each of the following would score 1 on the Imrie or modified Glasgow criteria:
   - WCC > 15 × 10^9/L.
   - Blood glucose > 10 mmol/L.
   - LDH > 600 iU/L.
   - Serum urea > 16 mmol/L.
   - PaO_2 < 8 kPa.
   - Calcium < 2 mmol/L.
   - Albumin < 32 g/L.

17 Upper GI

17.1 UPPER GI EMQs

1. For each of the following clinical scenarios please choose the most appropriate diagnosis. Each answer may be used once, more than once or not at all.

   Achalasia   Gastric ulcer
   Adenocarcinoma of the oesophagus   Hiatus hernia
   Biliary colic   Oesophageal varices
   Duodenal ulcer   Pancreatitis
   Gastric carcinoma   Squamous cell carcinoma of the
                                          oesophagus

   a. A 25-year-old female presents with difficulty swallowing liquids. She also complains of regurgitation of her evening meals, especially if she eats shortly before going to bed. She has noticed that she has lost some weight and has recently been treated for a chest infection.

   b. A 63-year-old woman with a 20-year history of heartburn is referred to you, as she is having trouble keeping on top of her symptoms despite taking 30 mg of lansoprazole every morning. She describes a feeling of acid coming up into her throat, which is worse at night. On examination you note that she is obese.

   c. A 57-year-old male comes to see you with his wife with recent onset of difficulty swallowing. He has noticed that it has been particularly difficult to eat his wife's Sunday roasts. He was diagnosed with GORD in his mid-20s and has been relatively asymptomatic on omeprazole since then. His wife is concerned that he has lost a stone in the past month.

2. For each of the following clinical scenarios please choose the most appropriate diagnosis. Each answer may be used once, more than once or not at all.

   Achalasia   Gastric ulcer
   Chronic pancreatitis   Indigestion
   Duodenal ulcer   Mallory–Weiss tear
   Duodenal lymphoma   Oesophageal carcinoma
   Gastric carcinoma   Oesophageal varices

a. A 70-year-old man attends the GP with a long history of pain in his upper abdomen, which comes on before meals when he is hungry. The pain does not radiate anywhere and is relieved by eating and by taking antacids. He has come to see you, as he is worried it might be something serious. He does not complain of any weight loss, and generally feels fit and well.

b. A 70-year-old man attends the GP with a long history of pain in his upper abdomen, which comes on before meals when he is hungry. The pain sometimes radiates to his back, and is lessened but not fully relieved by eating. He has been feeling tired lately and has lost around a stone in the last couple of months.

c. A 34-year-old female comes into hospital via the emergency department, following a prolonged episode of vomiting after a night of binge drinking, at the end of which she noticed some fresh blood in the vomit. She has since stopped vomiting and is feeling a bit better, but she is worried about the blood that she saw.

17.2 UPPER GI EMQ ANSWERS

1. a. Answer: Achalasia.

   This young lady has a typical presentation of achalasia, which tends to start with dysphagia to liquids and subsequently progresses to solids. Regurgitation of food at night is common due to pooling of food in the dilated oesophagus. Although she has lost some weight, which may cause concern about malignancy, her weight loss is far more likely to be a product of difficulty swallowing. Chest infections are common in patients with achalasia due to aspiration of regurgitated food particles.

   b. Answer: Hiatus hernia (sliding type).

   Although this lady is complaining of symptoms classical of GORD, it is likely that this is due to an underlying hiatus hernia, which is common in this age group and in overweight individuals. Sliding hiatus herniae are much more common than rolling hiatus herniae.

   c. Answer: Adenocarcinoma of the oesophagus.

   This gentleman has a long-standing history of GORD, which is a major risk factor for oesophageal cancer (adenocarcinoma over squamous cell). His weight loss and dysphagia on solids are worrying signs for an oesophageal malignancy. He needs an urgent gastroscopy (OGD) and staging investigations in order to assess if his disease is suitable for surgical resection.

2. a. Answer: Gastric ulcer.

   This man has symptoms classical of a gastric ulcer and is most likely "worried well" following his recent bereavement. However, given his age he should be referred for further investigations to exclude a more sinister pathology.

b. Answer: Gastric carcinoma.

These two questions show just how similar the histories of patients with gastric ulcers and carcinoma can be and are a reminder that all patients with these symptoms over the age of 55 years should be sent for further assessment with endoscopy.

c. Answer: Mallory–Weiss tear.

As she has been vomiting for a long time, she is most likely to have torn her lower oesophageal mucosa due to this. As the vomiting and bleeding were small volume and have since stopped, a variceal bleed is less likely. This woman should be reassured, advised about her alcohol drinking behaviours, and will require early OGD to ensure there is no more significant pathology.

17.3 UPPER GI SBAs

For each of the questions below, select the single best answer. Each option may be used once only.

1. A 32-year-old male with a known alcohol dependency presents following a 12-hour bout of repeated vomiting. He has now stopped being sick but is worried because he noticed some blood in his vomit on two occasions. Which of the following investigations is **not** indicated?
   a. Barium swallow.
   b. Clotting screen.
   c. Full blood count.
   d. Liver function tests.
   e. OGD.

2. Which of these is **not** a common cause of mechanical small bowel obstruction?
   a. Adhesions.
   b. Caecal carcinoma.
   c. Crohn's disease.
   d. Inguinal hernia.
   e. Post-operative ileus.

3. Which of the following is not indicated in the management of a sexually active female patient with right iliac fossa pain and tenderness?
   a. Abdominal ultrasound.
   b. Abdominal x-ray.
   c. Gynaecological and rectal internal examinations.
   d. MSU.
   e. Pregnancy test.

17.4 UPPER GI SBA ANSWERS

1. **Answer: Barium swallow.**

   This man is presenting with haematemesis, which may be due to a Mallory–Weiss tear. However with a history of alcohol dependency he may also have alcoholic liver disease, which can cause oesophageal varices. Because of this, liver synthetic and biochemical function tests (i.e. clotting screen and LFT) are warranted. A FBC should be performed to assess for pre-existing anaemia but may not indicate the severity of the bleed if it is very acute, and an OGD should be performed to look for varices. In this case a barium swallow would not tell us anything.

2. **Answer: Post-operative ileus.**

   Post-operative ileus is not a cause of mechanical obstruction; it is where the bowel stops functioning and is also known as 'paralytic ileus'. The others are all potential causes of mechanical bowel obstruction.

3. **Answer: Abdominal x-ray.**

   Plain abdominal x-ray is indicated in the investigation of abdominal pain to rule out obstruction, perforation or the presence of radio-opaque calculi; therefore given the history in this question, it is not warranted. The other four investigations, however, are appropriate given the history. Urinary tract infections and gynaecological disorders are common causes of right iliac fossa pain in young women, and so MSU, internal examinations, pregnancy test and USS are all indicated here.

18 Colorectal

18.1 COLORECTAL EMQs

1. For each of the following clinical scenarios please choose the most appropriate diagnosis. Each answer may be used once, more than once or not at all.

Acute appendicitis	Irritable bowel disease
Caecal adenocarcinoma	Infective colitis
Crohn's disease	Ischaemic colitis
Diverticular disease	Rectal adenocarcinoma
Familial adenomatous polyposis	Ulcerative colitis

a. A 15-year-old girl is brought to the emergency department by her parents. She was sent home from school due to feeling unwell and has been complaining of severe abdominal pain. She is tachycardic at 110 bpm, with respiratory rate of 22 and a blood pressure of 140/90 mmHg. Her temperature is 38°C. When you see her she is lying very still on the bed and looks flushed. She is very reluctant to let you examine her and is holding her right hip in flexion. Her white cell count is $19 \times 10^9/L$.

b. A 29-year-old female presents with a 6-month history of lethargy, malaise, vague abdominal pain and diarrhoea. She has lost about a stone in weight during this time despite the fact she has stopped going to the gym due to discomfort in her hips and lower back. She often gets mouth ulcers. On examination she has a tender fullness in the right iliac fossa.

c. An 18-year-old female is brought in by her mother who is concerned that her daughter has lost half a stone in weight over the past 2 months and has been complaining of abdominal pain that is interfering with her studies. She describes abdominal distension that is worse in the evenings and has recently been having a lot of diarrhoea, although denies any rectal bleeding. She has recently been accepted to Oxford University to read medicine. Physical examination is unremarkable. Stool sample, coeliac screen, FBC, LFT, ESR, CRP and ultrasound scan are all normal.

2. For each of the following clinical scenarios please choose the most appropriate diagnosis. Each answer may be used once, more than once or not at all.

Anal fissure   Diverticular bleed
Angiodysplasia   Diverticulitis
Colonic polyp   Haemorrhoids
Descending colon carcinoma   Rectal carcinoma
Diverticular abscess   Toxic megacolon

a. A 57-year-old obese male presents with a 3-day history of malaise, abdominal pain and low-grade fever. He denies any weight loss, rectal bleeding or change in bowel habit, although he tells you that he is prone to constipation. His father died of colorectal cancer at the age of 76. On examination he has guarding and marked tenderness over the left iliac fossa. His HR is 84 bpm, BP is 126/94 mmHg and temperature is 37.5°C.

b. A 57-year-old male attends the colorectal clinic on a 2-week wait referral from his GP. He has a 2-month history of bright red rectal bleeding that occurs with defecation. He denies change in bowel habit but describes a feeling of incomplete evacuation. On further questioning he has increasing fatigue and weight loss over recent weeks. His father had a stoma but he is unsure why.

c. A 47-year-old male with a long-standing history of constipation presents with pruritis ani and bright red rectal bleeding that occurs on the toilet paper following defecation. He denies pain on defecation, weight loss or change in bowel habit and is otherwise fit and well.

18.2 COLORECTAL EMQ ANSWERS

1. a. Answer: Acute appendicitis.
   This young girl has evidence of intra-abdominal sepsis and has a positive psoas sign. She most likely has acute, possibly perforated, appendicitis and should proceed to an appendicectomy.

   b. Answer: Crohn's disease.
   The gradual onset and pattern of this lady's symptoms suggest an inflammatory cause that, given the presence of mouth ulcers and a right iliac fossa mass, Crohn's disease is more likely than ulcerative colitis. The presence of a history of joint pain may indicate an underlying HLA-B27 genotype, which is common in this condition.

   c. Answer: Irritable bowel syndrome (IBS).
   IBS is a diagnosis of exclusion in the absence of any pathology or worrying features. This girl's symptoms appear to have presented during a time of stress, which is also typical of this disorder.

2. a. Answer: Diverticulitis.

This man has a classic history of diverticulitis and has many predisposing factors for diverticular disease, including obesity and a tendency to constipation. Absence of a palpable mass, swinging pyrexia or generalised peritonitis suggests that he is unlikely to have an abscess or acute perforation. Despite a family history of colorectal carcinoma, this is not a typical presentation; however he will require a colonoscopy after the inflammation has settled.

b. Answer: Rectal adenocarcinoma.

This gentleman has change in bowel habit with constitutional symptoms suggesting he may have cancer. He also describes tenesmus, suggesting he may have a rectal mass. Combined with the probable family history, rectal cancer is the most likely option and digital rectal examination may confirm a palpable mass.

c. Answer: Haemorrhoids.

This gentleman does not have any signs or symptoms of any sinister pathology. The preceding history of long-standing constipations means he is likely to have piles. The absence of pain on defecation rules out anal fissure as a cause.

18.3 COLORECTAL SBAs

For each of the questions below, select the single best answer. Each option may be used once only.

1. A 37-year-old female presents with bright red rectal bleeding that drips into the toilet after defecation. She is constipated and gets a sharp pain on opening her bowels that lasts for around 30 minutes. She denies weight loss and is otherwise fit and well.
   a. Anal cancer.
   b. Anal fissure.
   c. Haemorrhoids.
   d. Pilonidal sinus.
   e. Rectal prolapse.

2. You are the weekend doctor reviewing a patient with UC who has been receiving treatment for a flare for the last 2 weeks. He has developed worsening abdominal pain and distension over the past 24 hours and is beginning to show signs of shock. What is the most appropriate investigation you should perform?
   a. Abdominal radiograph.
   b. C-reactive protein.
   c. Flexible sigmoidoscopy.
   d. Full blood count.
   e. Stool culture.

18.4 COLORECTAL SBA ANSWERS

1. Answer: Anal fissure.

   Pain on defecations with bright red rectal bleeding is usually an anal fissure. Additionally, she is young and does not have any signs or symptoms of any sinister pathology. This is not a classical history of rectal prolapse or pilonidal sinus disease.

2. Answer: Abdominal radiograph.

   Whilst all of the answers are appropriate investigations to perform in a patient with a flare of UC, this patient is deteriorating and not responding to medical therapy. The concern is that he may have developed toxic megacolon. Flexible sigmoidoscopy should not be performed in this case, as there is an increased risk of perforation. The fastest and simplest way to confirm this diagnosis is a plain AXR. CT would also be an appropriate diagnostic test in this situation, as it would demonstrate dilatation of the colon as well as free air in the case of perforation, although it is not an option here. Additionally, AXR can be arranged quickly and can be interpreted by most clinicians in this setting.

Vascular

19.1 VASCULAR EMQs

1. For each of the following clinical scenarios please choose the most likely diagnosis. Each answer may be used once, more than once or not at all.

Acute embolic lower limb ischaemia   Fungal skin infection
Chronic lower limb ischaemia   Graft failure
Critical lower limb ischaemia   Lipodermatosclerosis
Deep vein thrombosis   Phlebitis
Diabetic foot   Uncomplicated varicose veins

a. A 69-year-old male with a PMH of AF presents to the emergency department with sudden onset of severe pain in his left leg. On examination the limb is cold and pale. He has no palpable popliteal or foot pulses in the left leg but good, strong pulses in the right. He is still able to move his leg and sensation is normal. What is the most likely diagnosis?

b. A 73-year-old male is referred with deformed feet. On examination his feet are warm and dry with bounding foot pulses. There is deformity of both feet with loss of the foot arches. He has ulceration between his toes and reduced sensation distally. What is the most likely diagnosis?

c. A 58-year-old woman presents itchy lower legs. She has a long history of varicose veins but has previously refused surgery. On examination she has significant varicosities affecting the long saphenous territory. These are associated with large, brown-pigmented, scaly patches above her medial malleolus that feel indurated on palpation. What is the most likely diagnosis?

19.2 VASCULAR EMQ ANSWERS

1. a. Answer: Acute embolic lower limb ischaemia.
   The short history and the presence of four of the 'six P's' (pulseless, pale, pain, perishingly cold) suggest the most likely diagnosis is acute lower limb ischaemia. This limb should still be considered salvageable at this point, and thus amputation is not appropriate; he will most likely need

surgical embolectomy. His AF is the most likely cause of his emboli, and hence he will need to be commenced on warfarin post-operatively.

b. Answer: Diabetic foot.

This description is of a Charcot foot with disorganisation of the foot joints and loss of the arches. Diabetics often have warm, dry feet with bounding foot pulses. Patients with Charcot feet have peripheral neuropathy; he has other evidence of this, i.e. painless ulceration on and loss of pain and temperature sensation.

c. Answer: Lipodermatosclerosis.

This lady has lipodermatosclerosis associated with venous insufficiency as a complication of her varicose veins. This is an uncommon complication characterised by eczema, itch, fat necrosis and pigmentation.

19.3 VASCULAR SBAs

For each of the questions below, select the single best answer. Each option may be used once only.

1. Which of the following is **not** part of the recommended management for a patient with a known abdominal aortic aneurysm?
   a. Annual ultrasound scan up to 7 cm diameter.
   b. Smoking cessation.
   c. Surgery if symptomatic.
   d. Surgery if the diameter is increasing by >0.5 cm per year.
   e. Use of statin therapy.

19.4 VASCULAR SBA ANSWERS

1. Answer: Annual ultrasound scan up to 7 cm diameter.

Biennial, not annual, surveillance with ultrasound scan is recommended up to 5.5 cm in diameter. Anything larger than this is an indication for elective repair.

20 Urology

20.1 UROLOGY EMQs

1. For each of the following clinical scenarios please choose the most appropriate diagnosis. Each answer may be used once, more than once or not at all.

Acute appendicitis	Pyelonephritis
Bladder stones	Testicular torsion
Cystitis	Torsion of testicular appendage
Epididymo-orchitis	Ureteric stones
Kidney stones	Urethritis

   a. A 23-year-old man presents with left-sided scrotal pain. The pain is severe and came on gradually over the course of the past 2 days. He describes some increased urinary frequency with mild dysuria. There is no history of haematuria or urethral discharge. He is sexually active and mentions that his most recent partner has recently been treated for an STI. He has had surgery for an undescended testis as a child.

   b. A 23-year-old man presents with a 4-hour history of left-sided scrotal pain. He was awoken in the night by the pain, which he describes as severe. The pain radiates to his right iliac fossa. He has a past medical history of an undescended testis as a child.

   c. An 11-year-old boy presents with a 6-hour history of a painful right testicle of sudden onset. On examination there is no swelling or erythema and the right testicle is of normal size and lie; however there is localised tenderness associated with a blue mark.

2. For each of the following clinical scenarios please choose the most appropriate diagnosis. Each answer may be used once, more than once or not at all.

Acute urinary retention	Ruptured abdominal aortic aneurysm
Bladder stone	Kidney stone
Chronic urinary retention	Pyelonephritis
Cystitis	Pyonephrosis
Hydronephrosis	Ureteric stone

a. A 25-year-old female presents with constant, severe left loin pain. This pain was preceded by a several-day history of dysuria and dull lower abdominal discomfort. Since developing the back pain she has been sweaty and has had two episodes of uncontrollable shaking. On examination she appears flushed, is tachycardic and pyrexial with a BP of 80/50 mmHg.

b. A 40-year-old man presents with acute onset of flank pain after lying in the garden all day. The pain is severe and radiates around his flank into the left side of his scrotum. He cannot get comfortable and is writhing around in discomfort. He has a tachycardia and is nauseated. He has a history of gout that is currently untreated.

c. A 75-year-old male presents to the emergency department with acute onset of severe left flank pain radiating to the back and collapse at home whilst digging in the garden. He has a tachycardia and is nauseated. His BP is 90/60 mmHg. He has a past medical history of hypertension is and is a smoker.

20.2 UROLOGY EMQ ANSWERS

1. a. Answer: Epididymitis.

   The gradual onset of testicular pain and the long duration points to an inflammatory condition rather than torsion. The association of lower urinary tract symptoms (LUTSs), such as frequency and dysuria, make epididymitis the likely diagnosis. The most likely infective organism in a man with epididymitis in this age group is *Chlamydia trachomatis*.

   b. Answer: Testicular torsion.

   Torsion of the testis should be at the top of the list of suspected causes of this man's pain given the sudden onset of severe pain and the short duration. The presence of lower abdominal pain is fairly typical, but means that other pathologies should be considered during the clinical evaluation (e.g. appendicitis, ureteric colic). Testicular torsion needs to be ruled out urgently in this situation due to the short window of time before the testicle infarcts.

   c. Answer: Torsion of testicular appendage.

   This young boy has torsion of the testicular appendage; however the presentation is often very similar to testicular torsion, and if there is any doubt, exploratory surgery should be performed to confirm the diagnosis.

2. a. Answer: Ureteric stone.

   This man has a typical presentation of ureteric colic that may be associated with his gout and may have been precipitated by dehydration. Obstruction of the tubular ureter causes colicky pain that radiates from the flank to the groin. There is associated microscopic haematuria due to trauma of the stone against the urothelium. He should be admitted for analgesia, IV fluid resuscitation and will need investigation with non-contrast CT scanning.

b. Answer: Pyelonephritis.

This woman has had simple cystitis for a couple of days but has now developed acute pyelonephritis due to haematological spread of infection. She has had two episodes of what sound like rigors and is likely to be very unwell due to sepsis. She should be admitted for IV fluid resuscitation and IV antibiotics.

c. Answer: Ruptured abdominal aortic aneurysm.

Sudden onset of flank pain in a patient of this age group should be treated as a leaking abdominal aortic aneurysm until proven otherwise. He should be treated with an ABCDE approach and fluid resuscitated. If the capabilities exist, he should undergo an emergency room USS to assess the diameter of the aorta. Laparotomy should not be delayed for CT scanning if the patient is unstable when a leaking AAA is suspected. Instead, urgent vascular surgical opinion should be sought.

20.3 UROLOGY SBAs

For each of the questions below, select the single best answer. Each option may be used once only.

1. A 76-year-old male has a 2-year history of difficulty passing urine. He describes having to wait for several seconds before initiation of his urinary stream, a poor stream and some terminal dribbling. He is usually up three or four times to pass urine during the night. He does not have any dysuria or haematuria. He takes ramipril for high blood pressure but is otherwise fit and well.

What is the most likely diagnosis?

a. Benign prostatic obstruction.

b. Bladder cancer.

c. Bladder stones.

d. Prostate cancer.

e. Renal stones.

2. A 17-year-old male presents with a 3-day history of gradual onset of scrotal pain and swelling. He complains of associated dysuria and penile discharge. What is the most likely causative organism?

a. *Escherichia coli*.

b. *Enterococcus faecal*.

c. *Klebsiella*.

d. *Neisseria gonorrhoeae*.

e. *Proteus mirabilis*.

3. Which type of calculi most commonly form staghorn calculi?

a. Calcium oxalate.

b. Cysteine.

    c. Purine.
    d. Struvite.
    e. Uric acid.

20.4 UROLOGY SBA ANSWERS

1. Answer: Benign prostatic hypertrophy (BPH).
   This is a typical presentation of BPH that is very common in older males. The haematuria at the start of the stream suggests a prostatic or urethral cause. The absence of systemic signs would suggest that this is not a cancer of the prostate, although this should be ruled out by histopathological analysis of tissue samples.

2. Answer: *Neisseria gonorrhoeae*.
   The history is suggestive of epididymo-orchitis, which is commonly caused by sexually transmitted infections in the younger age group (e.g. *Chlamydia trachomatis* and *Neisseria gonorrhoeae*). The other options would all be possible for a simple UTI.

3. Answer: Struvite.
   Struvite stones are a mixture of magnesium, ammonium and calcium phosphates and are the most common type of staghorn calculi. The often occur in the presence of chronic infection.

21 Trauma and burns

21.1 TRAUMA AND BURNS EMQs

1. For each of the following clinical scenarios please choose the most appropriate diagnosis. Each answer may be used once, more than once or not at all.

GCS 3	GCS 9
GCS 5	GCS 10
GCS 6	GCS 11
GCS 7	GCS 13
GCS 8	GCS 14

a. A 17-year-old male is brought into the emergency department at 10 p.m. on a Friday night following a fight after consuming 500 mL of neat vodka. A witness claims he was assaulted, sustaining several blows to the head. His RR is 14 breaths/minute, BP is 112/76 mmHg and HR is 94 bpm. He refuses to open his eyes and is unable to form coherent words, although he withdraws his finger upon contact with a neurotip. You wish to assess his disability status. What is his GCS?

b. A 78-year-old male who tripped and hit his head has been admitted for observation. He is usually fit and well and had remained conscious and oriented following the incident. Three hours after admission to the ward the nursing staff call you to review him as he has become drowsy. On examination he will open his eyes when you ask him and will generally obey commands; however he is no longer sure where he is or who you are. What is his GCS?

c. A 32-year-old male has been brought into the emergency department resus room following a road traffic accident where he was a front-seat passenger in a head-on collision. He was not wearing a seat belt and was thrown through the windscreen and onto the pavement. On arrival he is unconscious and there is no response to painful stimuli. What is his GCS?

21.2 TRAUMA AND BURNS EMQ ANSWERS

1. a. Answer: 7.

This young man is not opening his eyes (E = 1 out of 4) and is uttering incomprehensible sounds (V = 2 out of 5). However he is withdrawing from a painful stimulus (M = 4 out of 6). This gives him a GCS of 1 + 2 + 4 = 7.

   b. Answer: 13.

This man is opening his eyes to voice (E = 3 out of 4) and obeys commands (M = 5 out of 6) but is disoriented and confused (V = 4 out of 5). This gives him a current GCS of 13. He should have an urgent CT head, as he may have an evolving extradural haematoma leading to a reduction in his GCS. If an extradural haematoma is demonstrated, there should be discussion with neurosurgery for consideration of burr hole evacuation.

   c. Answer: 3.

This man scores the lowest possible scores for each component, which gives him a GCS of 3.

21.3 TRAUMA AND BURNS SBAs

For each of the questions below, select the single best answer. Each option may be used once only.

1. Which of the following organisms is most likely to be responsible for causing OSPI in a post-splenectomy patient?
   a. *Escherichia coli.*
   b. *Haemophilus influenzae.*
   c. *Pseudomonas aeruginosa.*
   d. *Staphylococcus aureus.*
   e. *Staphylococcus epidermidis.*

2. A 25-year-old female is brought into the emergency department following an RTA. Which of the following is usually treated conservatively?
   a. 2500 mL blood drained on insertion of a left-sided chest drain.
   b. Air under the diaphragm on CXR.
   c. Evidence of grade V splenic rupture on CT with a Hb of 5 g/dL despite continuous blood transfusion.
   d. Persistent BP of 85/60 mmHg despite appropriate fluid resuscitation.
   e. Suspected flail chest.

3. For which of the following presentations is a referral to a specialist burns unit not indicated?
   a. Burn to chest of an 8-year-old in the shape of an iron.
   b. Burn to forearm of a 5-year-old that is pink.

c. Burn to forearm of a 5-year-old that is white and charred.
d. Burn to forearm and hand of a 62-year-old woman with severe dementia.
e. Burn to lower limb from below knee to groin that is red and wet.

21.4 TRAUMA AND BURNS SBA ANSWERS

1. Answer: *Haemophilus influenzae.*
   overwhelming post-splenectomy infection (OPSI) is most commonly caused by encapsulated bacteria, such as *Haemophilus influenzae*, *Streptococcus pneumonia* and *Neisseria meningitids.*
2. Answer: Suspected flail chest.
   Although flail chest is a serious injury to sustain, in practice surgical intervention is not always necessary, as a combination of packing and strapping can achieve adequate outcomes without having to resort to major thoracic surgery. The other four scenarios are indication for immediate surgical exploration.
3. Answer: Burn to forearm of a 5-year-old that is pink.
   Unless the mechanism of injury was suspicious of a non-accidental injury, a superficial burn to the forearm of a 5-year-old child that is less than 5% TBSA is not an indication for referral to a specialist burn unit. Referral is indicated in any suspected cases of child abuse, special areas (including hands), large burns (more than 10% TBSA in an adult) and third-degree burns (where the burns are charred and white).

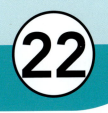

22 Post-operative care

22.1 POST-OPERATIVE CARE EMQs

1. For each of the following clinical scenarios please choose the single most likely diagnosis. Each answer may be used once, more than once or not at all.

Atelectasis	Pulmonary embolism
ARDS	Sepsis
Chest infection	SIRS
Haematoma	Subcutaneous abscess
MODS	Wound infection

a. You are called to see a 59-year-old female who is 1 day post-operative from a right mastectomy. She complains of discomfort across her right chest, which, on examination, is swollen and tense under the surgical wound. She appears pale and is slightly tachycardic. Her haemoglobin has dropped by 3 g/dL.

b. You are called to see a 75-year-old female who underwent a low anterior resection for rectal cancer 6 days ago. She has been complaining of pain in her left leg over the past couple of days and has been slow to mobilise. She suddenly has an episode of collapse with tachycardia, hypotension and tachypnoea.

c. You are called to see a 68-year-old male on the HDU who underwent an Ivor-Lewis oesophagectomy 2 days ago. He feels generally unwell but has no specific complaints. On reviewing his observation he has a temperature of 38.2°C, a HR of 95 bpm, BP is 110/75 mmHg and a RR of 22. His bloods are all within normal limits. On examination his wounds appear clean and dry, his chest is clear and his abdomen is soft. His urine is a bit cloudy in the catheter.

22.2 POST-OPERATIVE CARE EMQ ANSWERS

1. a. Answer: Haematoma.

   This patient has had a post-operative bleed causing blood to collect within the space created during surgery. Minor haematomas may be managed conservatively, but infected or large haematomas that exert pressure on the wound need to be drained and haemostasis achieved.

b. Answer: Pulmonary embolism.

This patient has several risk factors for VTE, including pelvic surgery, malignancy and immobility. She has been complaining of leg pain, which may suggest she had developed a DVT in that leg. The sudden respiratory and circulatory collapse should prompt immediate treatment with LMWH and subsequent confirmation of the diagnosis with CTPA. D-dimer in this patient is unlikely to be helpful, as it will be raised due to her recent surgery.

c. Answer: SIRS.

This man has three of the four criteria for SIRS, but no positive bacterial cultures at this time. He should be closely monitored with regular observations and should remain on the HDU, as this may be the beginning of sepsis. Blood and urine samples should be sent for culture.

22.3 POST-OPERATIVE CARE SBAs

For each of the questions below, select the single best answer. Each option may be used once only.

1. You are asked to review a post-operative patient who underwent a laparoscopic cholecystectomy 2 hours ago. She is complaining of severe abdominal pain, nausea and distension. The nursing staff have given her paracetamol and codeine as prescribed in the post-operative instructions. She has a past medical history of a perforated duodenal ulcer but has no known drug allergies. Which of the following analgesics would be the most appropriate?
   a. Diclofenac PR.
   b. Ibuprofen orally.
   c. Morphine orally.
   d. Morphine SC.
   e. Tramadol IV.

2. You review an elderly patient who underwent a complicated colonic resection with subsequent anastomotic leak that required him to undergo further laparotomy and formation of an end colostomy. He is now 7 days following his original operation and 2 days following the recent re-operation. He is still having problems with vomiting and his stoma has not started working. Regarding feeding, which of the following options is the most appropriate?
   a. Arrange for insertion of a central line and commence TPN.
   b. Arrange for insertion of NG tube and provide overnight NG feeds.
   c. Encourage oral intake with high-calorie diet.
   d. Prescribe oral nutritional supplements, e.g. Fortisips™.
   e. Take no action; his ileus is likely to settle within the next 24 hours.

3. Which of the following is not one of the SIRS criteria?
   a. Heart rate > 90.
   b. $PaCO_2 < 4.3$ kPa.
   c. Temperature < 36°C.
   d. WCC < 4×10^9/L.
   e. WCC > 15×10^9/L.

22.4 POST-OPERATIVE CARE SBA ANSWERS

1. Answer: Morphine SC.
   Both diclofenac and ibuprofen are NSAIDs that should not be administered to patients with a history of complicated ulcer disease. Both tramadol and codeine are weak opioids and should not be prescribed together. Using the WHO analgesia ladder, she should be prescribed a strong opiate, such as morphine. As she is nauseated, this should not be given orally, and SC is a common method of administrating morphine.

2. Answer: Arrange for insertion of a central line and commence TPN.
   This man has not had adequate nutrition for a week. Couple with his complicated post-operative course, he will be severely catabolic. He needs supplemental nutrition, and since his GI tract is currently non-functional, this should be via the parenteral route but should be converted to enteral as soon as possible.

3. Answer: WBC > 15×10^9/L.
   The definition of SIRS requires two or more of the following criteria to be present:
   - Temp > 38°C or < 36°C.
   - HR > 90 BPM.
   - RR > 20 breaths/minute or $PaCO_2 < 4.3$ kPa.
   - WCC > 12×10^9/L or < 4×10^9/L.

Index